James Meschter Anders

House-plants as sanitary Agents

Or, The Relation of growing Vegetation to Health and Disease.

James Meschter Anders

House-plants as sanitary Agents

Or, The Relation of growing Vegetation to Health and Disease.

ISBN/EAN: 9783337111397

Printed in Europe, USA, Canada, Australia, Japan

Cover: Foto ©ninafisch / pixelio.de

More available books at **www.hansebooks.com**

HOUSE-PLANTS AS SANITARY AGENTS;

OR, THE

RELATION OF GROWING VEGETATION TO HEALTH AND DISEASE.

COMPRISING ALSO A CONSIDERATION OF THE SUBJECT OF

PRACTICAL FLORICULTURE,

AND OF

THE SANITARY INFLUENCES OF FORESTS AND PLANTATIONS.

BY

J. M. ANDERS, M.D., Ph.D.,

LATELY LECTURER ON BOTANY IN THE WAGNER FREE INSTITUTE OF SCIENCE, MEMBER OF THE "BUREAU OF SCIENTIFIC INFORMATION," ACADEMY OF NATURAL SCIENCES, CHAIR OF FORESTRY AND THE RELATION OF PLANT LIFE TO HEALTH, ASSISTANT PHYSICIAN TO THE EPISCOPAL HOSPITAL, ETC.

PHILADELPHIA:
J. B. LIPPINCOTT COMPANY.
1887.

Copyright 1886 by J M. ANDERS.

PREFACE.

For the immense number of books published the present age is truly phenomenal. Among the various departments of medical literature, as well as those of the natural sciences, there are perhaps few subjects that have not found an author, while many have been treated of by numerous writers. If, then, it be considered excusable, on the one hand, for an author to offer to the world a new volume upon a subject already represented in our libraries by one or more excellent treatises, how much more readily will it be pardoned, on the other, for presenting to the public a branch of scientific literature which in the form of a book has not hitherto found an exponent.

Apart from the fact that our pathway has not been previously trodden, it has been owing largely to what the author ventures to hope may be regarded by the kind reader as new light which the pages of this little volume may shed upon a question of the greatest moment to every household, namely, how to improve the sanitary conditions of the home, that he has been able to persuade himself as to the advisability of undertaking the task of authorship. Let it be understood at the outset that this effort does not claim to be either a treatise upon hygiene or botany, the author's earnest wish being simply to set forth, in plain terms, the latest light regarding the effects of some of the various physiological functions in plants and flowers upon the atmosphere in general, and the air of dwellings in particular, as well as the application of this knowledge to the laws of health.

Most of the subjects treated in this volume have formed the bases of papers previously published, at greater or lesser intervals, in sundry periodicals. Though neither in their original form nor sequence, these articles, after some elaboration, are now offered collectively with some additional facts.

As will appear in the succeeding pages, most of the conclusions put forward have been arrived at from the results of an almost continuous series of personal experiments extending over a period of eight years.

The chief purpose of the writer will have been accomplished if he succeeds in proving that plants and flowers, particularly when cultivated in-doors, are worthy to be placed in the foremost rank of sanitary agencies.

The mass of evidence at hand relating to the subject in the author's opinion establishes the complete efficacy of living plants as preventive measures in that deadly malady, consumption of the lungs, as well as the signal services they are capable of rendering in certain other conditions of disease.

Still another motive actuating the author has been an ardent desire to render more intense and widespread a popular love for plants and flowers, and to aid in creating a public sentiment which would result in rendering their cultivation more general. While the subjects discussed within its pages are, without a single exception, of a scientific character, the work is intended not only for professional readers, but also for the already large and constantly-increasing element of the lay population who are turning their attention to the pursuit of popular scientific knowledge.

Owing to the engrossing character of his professional duties as a practising physician, the author has been obliged to prepare the pages of this volume partly during short intervals of leisure and partly under the glare of the midnight lamp, which facts must serve as his apology for any shortcomings.

To Professor Thomas Meehan the author owes sincere thanks for having written the admirable chapter on "Practical Floriculture;" and also to Mr. Howard S. Anders for the careful manner in which he prepared the index.

The concluding chapters treat of the sanitary influences of forest-growth,—a subject engrossing, and deservedly so, a large share of the attention of scientific observers.

1529 NORTH EIGHTH STREET, PHILADELPHIA, September, 1886.

TABLE OF CONTENTS.

CHAPTER I.
PAGE

. The material relations of plant life to man recognized from the remotest antiquity—Plants prized by the ancients for their beauty and perfume—Historical sketch of their use as objects of decoration—Poetic allusions to Empire Flora—Living plants formerly regarded as unwholesome in sleeping-rooms—Plants not tolerated in the sick-chamber in past time—Funereal plants of the ancient Greeks and Romans—Subsequent departure from the opinion that plants have an injurious effect—Recent progress and the aim of Sanitary Science 13

CHAPTER II.

Organic functions—Their analogies—The older views upon plant respiration—Assimilation—Its effect upon the air—Respiration—Its permanence—Its effects—Too slight to prove deleterious—Von Pettenkofer's dictum—Uniformity of the amount of carbon dioxide and oxygen in the air—Experiments in the Royal Winter Garden in Munich—Plant-breathing no valid objection to growing plants in the living- and sleeping-rooms—Absorption of moisture from the air by the leaves of plants—Only possible when the roots are not supplied with enough moisture—Experiments adduced . . 29

CHAPTER III.

House-plants and malaria—Brief description of malaria—Intermittent and remittent types—Dumb ague—The cause a specific ferment—Is not the result of organic decomposition—The conditions essential to the production of malaria—The possibility of house-plants causing malaria, and how this can be averted—The victims of malaria—Effect of odorous emanations—Most of them delightful—A few of them only are injurious—The scent of roses—Objections to living plants within dwellings answered 55

CHAPTER IV.

Hygienic influences of house-plants—Transpiration—Experiments showing its rate, etc.—Effect of transpiration on the dew-point—Table of results—Summary of investigations—Effect of anatomical formation of leaves upon the rate of transpiration—The solar rays the chief exciting cause—Other modifying influences—Obvious effect of transpiration to increase the proportion of moisture in closed rooms—Experiments at the Episcopal Hospital, Philadelphia—Their results proving the ability of plants to increase the degree of humidity of living-rooms—The air of living-rooms also shown to be dryer than the outer air, especially when heated by the hot-air furnace—The effects of transpiration in lowering the temperature—The quantity of atmospheric moisture essential to health—The effect of temperature and relative humidity upon the rate of evaporation from our bodies—Small fluctuations in temperature and degree of saturation of vital moment to preserve health—Moisture furnished by plants highly serviceable where dry furnace heat is employed—The evil effects of furnace heat pointed out—Its relation to bodily ills—Plants becoming the means of obviating distressing symptoms—The high rank taken by plants and flowers as sanitary agencies 76

CHAPTER V.

Ozone—General statements relating thereto—Various modes of generating ozone—Do plants possess the power to generate it?—Experimental investigation of the question—Description of the tests for ozone—The first observations conducted in Horticultural Hall, Fairmount Park, Philadelphia—Description of same—Later experiments with glass case—In-door and out-door experiments with odorous and non-odorous flowers—Conclusions drawn from the results obtained—A reinvestigation of the subject—Similar methods employed—The results with the flowers identical—Experiments with odorous foliage—Interesting results from the use of pine foliage—The nature of this ozone-generating process discussed—Facts and experiments by others corroborating our own conclusions—Sanitary value of ozone—Value of flowering plants as purifiers of the air of dwellings, which is usually abominable—Sources of house-air impurities—House-plants as health-giving agents—Moral influences of plants and flowers—Review of sanitary relation of growing plants—Amount of plant life necessary for ordinary sanitary purposes 112

CHAPTER VI.

House-plants as sanitary agents in the sick-room—Their effect to prevent the transmission of communicable diseases—Their value in acute febrile diseases, and especially during the convalescence from the latter—Hygienic importance of the Solarium in hospitals—House-plants especially valuable in the chambers of chronic invalids—Their therapeutic application in functional nervous disorders—In inflammation of the throat—In true croup—In acute and chronic bronchitis and laryngitis—Description of different forms of chronic bronchitis—Advantages of growing plants in their treatment—Proportion of plants required—The value of living plants as preventives of bronchitis 153

CHAPTER VII.

Living plants useful in consumption of the lungs—The latter disease very fatal, though not universally so—General facts relating to its etiology—Experiments tending to show its communicability from person to person—Professor R. Koch's discovery of the bacillus tuberculosis, which is the specific organism causing phthisis—His researches show that phthisis is infectious—Conditions under which the bacillus develops are peculiar—Treatment of phthisis discussed—No antidote to the bacillus found as yet—House-plants especially valuable in preventing the destructive work of this organism—Supporting evidence of a practical kind—The author's observations among florists—Cases confirmatory recorded by other writers—Requisites of health resorts for consumptives—Advantages of a home sanitarium—The relative amount of plant-growth required—The value of growing plants in confirmed phthisis—Cases illustrating the utility of plants in confirmed phthisis . . . 174

CHAPTER VIII.

Soil for potting flowers—It should be composed of decaying sods—It should be porous—Fertilizers—They should be well decayed—Plants requiring special soils—Chemical fertilizers—Heat and moisture—Continuous supply of moisture to the roots generally necessary—The proper temperature variable—Plants that love light and warmth, and those loving shade—Air of living-rooms congenial to most plants—Roots love darkness—Feeding roots keep near the surface of the soil—Watering of plants—This supplies oxygen—Sulphurous gases injurious—Temperature of water—

Potting—Necessity of holes for drainage—Cuttings—Training of plants—New varieties from seed—Insects and disease—The window-garden—Flowers suited to in-door cultivation—Aquariums—The greenhouse conservatory—Designs for the latter—Methods of heating—Out-door gardening—Rosery 209

CHAPTER IX.

Devastation of primitive forests—Evil results from—Conservative influence of forests on the moisture of the soil—Forests feed streams and springs—Relation of forest-growth to malaria—Effects of Eucalyptus plantations upon malaria—Vegetable mould, its advantages and disadvantages—Chemico-vital action of woods—Their mechanical influence to prevent malaria—Forests as preventives of cholera—Their climatic effects—The protective influence of trees by opposing wind-currents—Happy influence of the woodland upon extremes of temperature—The forest air cooler in summer than the open air—Effects of the delicious coolness of shade—Action of woods on the temperature of the air in winter—Their influence upon the humidity of the air—Chiefly due to transpiration—Experiments related—Forest moisture more uniform than that from other sources—Its effects in impeding radiation at night—Experiments by Tyndall—Effects of woods upon the rainfall—Forests as natural ozone producers—Coniferæ develop ozone actively—Object of wild-flowers in nature—Climatic effects of forests local in character 257

CHAPTER X.

Natural tendency after clearing to replace old with new forest species—Difference between native species of the Atlantic and Pacific coasts—Their adaptation to conditions of soil and climate—Best proportion of woodland for sanitary objects—The forests of the United States—They need not now excite grave apprehension—Need of better management of our forests—Arbor-day—Æsthetic influences of the woodland flora—The sanitary effects of forests—Their value at health stations—Forest air beneficial in the treatment of bronchial affections and phthisis—Climatic requisites for pulmonary invalids—The equable humidity of forests not objectionable—The advantages of pine-groves to the consumptive—Commoner forms of phthisis briefly described—The proper forest area adapted to their treatment—Suitable localities for winter and summer forest resorts—Hygienic influences of city parks—Kinds of trees for planting in streets and public parks . 303

HOUSE-PLANTS AS SANITARY AGENTS;

OR, THE

RELATION OF GROWING VEGETATION
TO HEALTH AND DISEASE.

CHAPTER I.

The material relations of plant life to man recognized from the remotest antiquity—Plants prized by the ancients for their beauty and perfume—Historical sketch of their use as objects of decoration—Poetic allusions to Empire Flora—Living plants formerly regarded as unwholesome in sleeping-rooms—Plants not tolerated in the sick-chamber in past time—Funereal plants of the ancient Greeks and Romans—Subsequent departure from the opinion that plants have an injurious effect—Recent progress and the aim of Sanitary Science.

INTRODUCTION.

SINCE plant life, from the advent of man upon the earth, has been accessible to him, it may reasonably be inferred that from the highest antiquity many important relations of vegetation to his various needs have been recognized. So illustrious a savant as Linnæus remarked, "Plants must have yielded man his earliest food, his first-built habitations; his utensils and his weapons must alike have been derived from the same source." Further than merely to make mention of such material relations to plants as affect either the productive resources of a region or the various domestic, artistic, and industrial purposes to which they are put, would seem to be somewhat irrelevant to our present purpose. It should be remarked, however, that the important rôle which plants perform in maintaining the harmonious composition of our atmosphere, as well as the task imposed upon them of preparing all animal food which they elaborate from the mineral substances, have been long since among the most familiar facts in natural science. Than such general considerations alone furnish there could, perhaps, be no more convincing evidence of man's intimate relation with the vegetable kingdom. *Apropos* of the well-known metaphor (old) "mother earth," the observation of Professor von Pettenkofer relating thereto is worthy of note, since it admirably serves to point out a truth frequently overlooked, to wit: "Since the vegetable world comes between us" (referring to man and the earth or mineral kingdom), "we should rather call earth our grandmother than our mother." The truth of this statement becomes plainly evident when we reflect that our food is derived either directly from vegetable life or indirectly from the same source, as when obtained from animals which feed upon vegetable structures; while on the other hand plants are entirely nourished by inorganic matter, and hence the mineral being farther removed from us by one generation than the vegetable kingdom, we should naturally have a greater feeling of affection for the latter than the former. At all events, we cannot deny our obligations to the vegetable world any more than we can deny our sacred obligations to our nearest of kin.

It is well known that the greater number of the more important substances which go to make up the physician's armamentarium are of vegetable origin. Notwithstanding the fact that our most salutary remedies are extracted from vegetable tissues, growing plants, particularly when cultivated in-doors, have not, until within recent years, been regarded as possessing therapeutic or hygienic advantages. Though known to be actively carried on, their vital functions did not appear to attract the attention of sanitarians, excepting when according as they were placed, *e.g.*, in sleeping-apartments or the sick-chamber, they were considered to be positively deleterious to health. It should be kept in remembrance that not only the laity were deeply imbued with the seriousness of this old-time superstition, but also our most illustrious authors spoke in vigorous terms against their cultivation under the circumstances above named. Despite, however, the universality of this ancient idea, which in great measure debarred growing plants from the living-apartments, they have in all ages been highly prized for their beauty and sweet perfume. . They likewise have been and still are utilized as the chief objects of ornamental decoration on all occasions of public festivity. Under such circumstances, when tastefully grouped, one hears only encomiums upon the beauty and variety of forms presented by such a galaxy of plants and flowers. The introduction of these elaborate decorations occurred about the year 1867, when, so says the *Court Journal,* Sir Edward Scott had the first grand floral ball in Grosvenor Square. The order to a well-known florist was that he (Sir Edward) wished his to be the handsomest ball of the season, and that he would place his house in the hands of the florist for three days to do as he liked, regardless of expense. The decorations caused a perfect furore, and it was the means of entirely revolutionizing the style of artistic decorations, not only in London, but also in every part of the United Kingdom, and, indeed, the whole of Europe and America. Moreover, this pleasant innovation had the happy effect of proving for all future time an incentive to the more general cultivation of plants. It is most gratifying to be able to note that the popularity of the practice has been growing to the present time, shedding a beneficent influence upon the progress of social refinement. In the light of modern investigation, however, it would surely be rash to continue to hold the once popular view that the main purpose of plants and flowers is to appeal to our sense of the beautiful as displayed in their colors and varied forms. This statement will become clear to the mind of the reader, provided we shall be able to make good our promise to show that whilst remarkable for their beauty they are not less remarkable for their effects upon human health, or, in other words, to establish new and vital relations between vegetable growth and the human family.

According to Pouchet ("The Universe," p. 259), the ancients had their "coronary plants:" these were consecrated to Venus, and at feasts each guest wore a chaplet. It is certain, therefore, that the notion which ascribed to Empire Flora baneful influences was neither held because plants in rooms were not greatly admired, nor because their presence gave no pleasure. To show the value of plants as educators, ample testimony is afforded by the ancient Jewish writers, whose teachings drawn from floral life abound in lessons of great worth.

The many allusions to plants and flowers, and the numerous floral similes found in Holy Writ, cannot fail to convince any reasonable mind that a passion for flowers was firmly rooted in the minds of the ancient Hebrews. It has been stoutly contended by the *Jewish World* that the passion for flowers is eminently Eastern. The Persian, for instance, will to this day sit before his favorite flower in mute adoration, on pleasant thoughts intent, apparently deriving great pleasure from its gay colors and graceful forms.

The poet has ever taken numerous and among them many of his happiest metaphors from the realms of the floral empire. As has been truly remarked, there are few poets, if any, who, when inspired by beautiful spring, do not introduce references to blooming vegetation.

> "Spring, Summer, Autumn: of all three,
>   Whose reign is loveliest there?
> Oh! is not she who paints the ground
> When its frost-fetters are unbound,
>   The fairest of the fair?
>
> "I gaze upon her violet beds,
>   Laburnums golden-tress'd,
> Her flower-spiked almonds; breathe perfume
> From lilac and syringa bloom,
> And cry, I love Spring best!"
>   Mrs. Southey.

In an expressive couplet, Shakespeare has, in his vision, associated some of the charms of plant life with dreary winter:

"But flowers distill'd, though they with winter meet,
Lose but their share, their substance still lives sweet."

So the following verses, alike pleasing and soulful, of our own revered countryman, doubly illustrious as poet and prose writer, Dr. Oliver Wendell Holmes, may not be amiss:

"Her hands are cold, her face is white;
No more her pulses come and go;
Her eyes are shut to life and light;
Fold the white vesture, snow on snow,
And lay her where the violets blow.

"If any, born of kindlier blood,
Should ask, what maiden lies below?
Say only this: a tender bud,
That tried to blossom in the snow,
Lies withered where the violets blow."

Let it therefore be distinctly understood that the love of plants and flowers has, according to the records of ancient history, always existed in the hearts and minds of most persons; and though, as already intimated, they were very commonly banished from living-apartments in the past, this innate affection has during all the ages defied the assaults of this baseless prejudice. When we regard the foregoing facts, it is not a little surprising that these frequently indispensable floral treasures could even have been supposed to exercise hurtful effects, and in consequence to have been practically denied admission to the household upon ordinary occasions. It remains to be said to their credit, however, that the opinions of our predecessors upon this point were fostered by the teachings of the leading authorities of their day and generation.

It was popularly held in former times, especially by the laity, that plants in sleeping-rooms were particularly unwholesome; and, although shown to be erroneous, this old idea is in some quarters still adhered to with remarkable pertinacity. But this popular fallacy was not so ill founded as some others, it having been chiefly based upon the function of respiration in plants, which function consists, as is well known, in abstracting oxygen from and returning to the atmosphere carbon dioxide; the former substance being needful to animal respiration, while the presence of the latter, even in small per centum, is highly pernicious in its effects upon health. Hence it is clear that, should plants through this function have any perceptible influence upon the atmosphere, they must prove to be correspondingly unwholesome. As will appear evident hereafter, the excellent investigations of Professor von Pettenkofer into this subject leave no room for doubt that this objection which has been urged against the presence of growing plants in bed-chambers is practically groundless.

To confirm fully the unity of opinion that has prevailed both in Europe and America concerning the supposed injurious effects of living plants when kept in the sleeping-rooms, the following brief citations are here presented. The *London Medical Record*, 1880, has the following statement: "There was once—still is, perhaps—a superstition that plants and flowers are unwholesome," etc. In his excellent work on Practical Floriculture,* Mr. P. Henderson, in reply to the question so frequently raised, namely, Are plants injurious to health? remarks in the first place, that if physicians are asked the same question, three out of six will reply that they are. He continues, "They will generally follow up the reply by a learned disquisition on horticultural chemistry; will tell you that at night plants give out carbonic acid gas, which is poison to animal life, and consequently if we sleep in a room where plants are kept we of necessity inhale this gas and sickness will follow. No theory can be more destitute of truth. That plants give out carbonic acid gas is certain, but that it is given out in quantities sufficient to affect our health in the slightest degree is utter nonsense."

The *London Globe* of recent date is authority for the statement that "not so very many years ago the danger of keeping such things (plants) in a bedroom was a good deal pooh-poohed by practical persons, who regarded the stories told in that connection as old women's tales belonging to the same category as the myth about sleeping under the moon or taking a siesta under a yew-tree." While the writer is not prepared to deny the above historical statement, he must confess to an inability, after a careful search through the meagre literature of the subject, to find anything tending to support the idea sanctioning the cultivation of plants in bedrooms.

The following extract from the same article relates

---

* This work, it should be remarked, was published in 1878.

directly to the point under consideration: "But then there were published terrible accounts of fair dames who, despising the warnings in question and depositing bouquets or flower-pots in their rooms at night, had met with a fate almost as tragic as that in the doleful ballad of 'The Mistletoe Bough.' Thereupon the scientific world, with the whole crew of unlearned folk at its heels, rushed to the opposite conclusion, and adopted a theory that illness and even death might result from sleeping in an apartment adorned with living plants or fresh cuttings."

Nor did our ancestors tolerate the practice of keeping plants in the sick-chamber. The universality of this popular prejudice can be attested by some distinguished writers. An eminent physician and well-known writer upon medical subjects, Dr. Hiram Corson, of Conshohocken, Pennsylvania, contributed an interesting paper to the *Norristown Herald* of December 2, 1881, in which, regarding the point in question, the following expressive statement occurs: "During the last half-century, how much longer I know not, the universal idea of lay people and physician has been that it was injurious to health to have growing plants in a sick-chamber. Physicians were earnest in their disapproval of having them in rooms occupied by the sick or the invalid. From my own observation during many years, I believe that not more than one in ten but advised against them. Indeed, I never knew of a single one who gave approval of such a course. So current was the belief of their injurious tendency that the question was not put to the physician at all." The explanation of this belief having become so firmly established in the minds of all, not excepting the most learned sanitarians of former ages, is not, perhaps, so apparent. Setting aside the unfounded reasons above given for excluding them from the sleeping- and living-rooms in general, there is no valid objection to their presence in the sick-room anywhere discoverable in the scant literature upon the subject, except in the case of plants emitting offensive odors. The prevalent idea among our forefathers as to their unwholesomeness in the sick-room must therefore be considered to be worthy of a place in the category of popular traditions, and in the present instance each succeeding generation has, for an indefinite period, copied and tenderly embraced the notion as a sacred legacy to be carefully and religiously preserved.

The ancient theory that the vital functions carried on by the animal and vegetable worlds are really antagonistic should, in view of the present state of scientific knowledge, be peremptorily abandoned. No task has been found beset with greater difficulties, however, than to dislodge from the minds of the general public an inherited dogma, be it never so gratuitous or fallacious. Though growing plants were formerly rigidly excluded from the sick-room, where their cheering influence alone would have been capable of great good to the sick, it is interesting to observe that in antiquity the Greeks and Romans had a certain blind or superstitious faith in their so-called "funereal plants," the history of which has been developed in a very interesting way by G. A. Langguth in his "Antiquatis Feralium apud Græcos et Romanos," Lipsiæ, 1738.

It is worthy of note that each plant had a certain mission to fill, and the author traces their employment from the commencement of the malady to the close of the funeral ceremonies. "When the malady began to alarm a family seriously, they suspended at the patient's door boughs of the favorite tree of Apollo, the inventor of medicine, in order to secure a favorable turn to the complaint. To the branches of laurel were added tufts of the Rhamnus, consecrated to Janus, and which was supposed to preserve the dwelling from all harm. But if, despite this invocation for aid, death overtook the sick person, they substituted for these plants black boughs of cypress, the emblem of Pluto and Proserpine, or branches of larch, the funereal tree, as Pliny calls it." Although the above may be regarded as a true picture of Roman and Greek customs, it will also serve as a beautiful illustration of the extravagant theories of ancient mythology, which we find additionally credited trees with marvellous powers, such as their being the abode of spirits both sacred and demoniac. Plants, particularly trees, were supposed to be sentient beings, and even possessed of souls. In this age of enlightenment, strange as it may appear, some relics of these ancient superstitions still linger in certain quarters of our globe. Obviously, it would be eminently undesirable that our ideas should revert to the notions held in the days of these fictitious legends.

The foregoing views, which unanimously concur that plants exercise an insalutary effect upon the atmosphere of occupied apartments, prevailed very generally down to about the year 1875, after which period there began to be a gradual departure from this view, opinions now becoming divided, a few writers contending that they are innocuous. There soon followed a lively controversy, particularly as to the practice of keeping plants and flowers in bedrooms and the sick-chamber, which controversy was not without good effects, since those who engaged in it brought common sense and reason to bear upon the question. Certain acute observers also came to realize that practical experience could furnish us no arguments opposed to the opinion that plants even at night have no appreciable deleterious effect. There were still others who were so fortunately circumstanced as to have the opportunity of drawing upon their own personal experience to assist them to clear up the question. Thus at about this period Mr. Henderson, in his "Practical Floriculture" (*loc. cit.*), wrote as follows: "No healthier class of men can be found than greenhouse operatives, which makes me sometimes think that plants have a health-giving effect rather than otherwise. But doctors may tell us that our workmen are only at work in the daytime, and that it is at night that their carbonic acid is emitted. Here we meet them by the information that in most cases the gardener in charge of greenhouses often has to be up the greater part of the night in winter, and the greenhouse, from its warmth, is universally taken as his sitting-room, and sometimes as his bedroom; such was my own experience for three winters. I had charge of a large amount of glass, situated nearly a mile from my boarding-house, too far to go and come at midnight, with the thermometer below zero. Our means of heating were entirely inadequate, so that the fires had to be looked to every three or four hours. Disregarding all my kind-hearted employer's admonitions, I nightly slept on the floor of the hothouse, which was rank with tropical growth. The floor was just the place to inhale the gas, if there had been much to inhale. It did not hurt me, however, and has not yet, and that is a score of years ago."

In 1877, Professor von Pettenkofer published an account of his experiments upon the "Hygienic Influence of Plants" (*Popular Science Monthly*, December, 1878), in which he clearly showed that plants in rooms were, leaving out of consideration special cases, incapable of hurtful effects. These investigations will elsewhere be fully detailed. Already one year previous to the appearance of the article of Professor von Pettenkofer the author had published the results of an experimental study of the function of transpiration ("Transpiration of Plants," *American Naturalist*, November, 1877), which investigations, though they did not anticipate any of the conclusions advanced by Von Pettenkofer in his paper, did nevertheless, as will be seen hereafter, anticipate a change of opinion respecting the influence of growing plants on the atmosphere of closed apartments; the latter inference naturally growing out of the remarkable fact shown by these experiments, namely, that the amount of moisture exhaled is so greatly in excess of what had been thought to be the usual quantity that the degree of humidity of an enclosed space desirable could thereby be regulated.

It is interesting to note that about the time when

Von Pettenkofer published the article before referred to, in which he exploded the theory of the injuriousness of plants from the function of respiration, the investigations of the writer directed public attention to the fact that plants, through the function of transpiration, are capable of exerting sanitary influences upon the atmosphere of dwellings. *As to the exactness of this statement,* however, the gentle reader shall be invited to pass dispassionate judgment.

Since then the subject has been attracting a large share of attention, not only in America but also on the part of transatlantic scientists; but as these more recent facts relating to the literature of our theme will be brought out in the discussion to follow, to review them here would be supererogatory.

Since vegetable life constitutes so great a factor in the organic world, a thorough study of the vital functions of plants seems to be almost an imperious necessity.

Exact knowledge pertaining to some of the more occult physiological processes has of late been rapidly unfolding. Again, as our knowledge in this direction increases, we shall the more readily acknowledge how much we owe to vegetation, for it cannot be gainsaid that our love for and appreciation of plants and flowers must, to a great extent, go hand in hand with the increase in our knowledge concerning their influence upon our health and welfare. It will appear hereafter that the salient practical points to be discussed in the following pages are closely connected with many of the leading principles of the science of health.

Than hygiene there has, within the last decade, been

no other science more progressive, and surely none is of more signal importance alike to the medical fraternity and the general public. It may be not amiss to note, *en passant*, that its rapid development has not been owing solely to the labors of medical men, but it can justly arrogate to itself the honor of having engaged the attention of some of the ablest minds outside the medical profession.

Though sanitary science does not aim to investigate the etiology of disease, it is safe to assume that a large per centum of many of the most fatal as well as the most common ills could, by proper attention to the known laws of health, be prevented, and it will not be denied that such a course would be a means of escaping many diseases of whose causes we are as yet in utter ignorance.

There is among lay people still universal need of a better knowledge of sanitary matters; and in the department of this science known as domestic hygiene, which embraces the topics, food, raiment, the air of the home, etc., more popular knowledge is urgently needful. So that, in view of the above statements, the facts hereafter put forward will, it is hoped, show not only that these "jewels of heaven's own setting" are not merely to be held as "a source of pleasure conveying a gleam of sunshine into millions of homes," but also that they possess well-proven hygienic influences upon the atmosphere in general and that of living-apartments in particular.

Having briefly overlooked the old views respecting the sanitary relations of plants and flowers, and having shown that professional as well as in a great measure the current of popular opinion has of late years undergone a marked change, the author purposes in the two succeeding chapters to present in detail the reasons and scientific data upon which this reversion of verdict has been based.

CHAPTER II.

Organic functions—Their analogies—The older views upon plant-respiration—Assimilation—Its effect upon the air—Respiration—Its permanence—Its effects—Too slight to prove deleterious—Von Pottenkofer's dictum—Uniformity of the amount of carbon dioxide and oxygen in the air—Experiment in the Royal Winter Garden in Munich—Plant-breathing no valid objection to growing plants in the living- and sleeping-rooms—Absorption of moisture from the air by the leaves of plants—Only possible when the roots are not supplied with enough moisture—Experiments adduced.

In a general way, it may be said, the physiology of the vegetable kingdom does not materially differ from that of the animal. Like animals, plants possess such functions as assimilation, absorption, transpiration, respiration, circulation, secretion, reproduction, and so on. Although having many important functions in common, that there are exhibited, as formerly held, some apparent functional contrasts between the vegetable and animal worlds will not be denied; but to contend that the functions of the one operate to any extent injuriously upon the health and well-being of the members of the other cannot by known facts be proved beyond question. In his lectures delivered during several years before the Park Museum of Natural History, Claude Bernard first pointed out the resemblances between the physiological processes of the two organic kingdoms, thereby making the scientific world his eternal debtor. By his ingenious and not less delicate experiments upon the glycogenic function of the liver, he conclusively showed that sugar, which is so important a principle in vegetable sap, is formed in this organ. The effect of his tracing their functional analogies has been to produce a change of scientific opinion upon this important subject. It may be safely assumed that whenever the vegetable seem to differ fundamentally from the animal functions, or, in other words, when the former seem to pursue opposite directions, it will be found on looking deeper that in reality the diversions are neither more nor less than salutary,—interventions designed by the author of nature to repair certain disturbances effected by the animal kingdom. Though the means are at variance, they yet work beautifully together to an harmonious end. In this connection, we are more especially concerned with but three of the organic functions above named,—to wit, assimilation, absorption, and respiration.

The teaching of the older botanists was that during darkness respiration in plants is exactly opposed to their diurnal breathing; that is to say, in nocturnal respiration plants are giving off carbon dioxide and taking from the atmosphere oxygen, whereas in diurnal they give to the atmosphere large amounts of oxygen and rid it of carbon dioxide. It was further taught that plants under the influence of light pour into the air vastly more oxygen than they abstract during the night; also that they absorb from it much more carbon dioxide each day than they produce at night. In this manner they explained the important office on the part of plant life to maintain the harmonious composition of the atmosphere. While it is true that to the vegetable world is confided the trust just stated, the above explanation in the light of subsequent researches is really incorrect. The interchange of gases so rapidly carried on during the day, consisting, as already intimated, in withdrawing carbon dioxide from the air and emitting oxygen in abundance, is not a respiratory phenomenon, but it is to be properly regarded as the act of assimilation, which function is solely dependent upon the influence of sunlight and hence occurring only during the day, in all parts of the plant containing chlorophyll. It would, perhaps, be irrelevant to give here a statement of the various processes concerned in assimilation. It should, however, be remarked that in all green or chlorophyll-bearing portions of the plant carbon dioxide and water are decomposed, and from their component elements compounds of carbon and hydrogen (carbohydrates) are formed. To pursue the consideration a single step further, it may be said that compounds rich in oxygen are taken into the plant, peroxide of hydrogen, carbon dioxide, and water, for example. In their excellent "Text-Book of Botany" Prantl and Hyrtl have pointed out a well-known and important botanical fact, namely, that assimilated substances which are formed from the compounds derived from without are very poor in oxygen, hence it naturally follows that during the act of assimilation a considerable portion of the oxygen absorbed in a combined form must be liberated and evolved by the plants.

Than to estimate the amount of oxygen which plants at every stomata distil into the atmosphere, nothing can be more simple; and Pouchet ("The Universe," p. 295) gives us an account of this beautiful experiment. It is only necessary to put the plant to be experimented with under a bell-glass filled with water, and as soon as it is exposed to the light all its foliage becomes covered with bubbles of gas, which are disengaged from it and rise without ceasing to the top of the water. If we now analyze the product collected there, we find from the brilliancy it gives to bodies in a state of ignition that it is oxygen and in possession of all its attributes. It is therefore to the emission of oxygen during the process of assimilation, which, by the older botanists, was ignorantly considered to be plant-breathing, that we are to ascribe the happy effect of plants upon the atmosphere whereby this medium is kept in a condition suited to animal respiration. If, then, it be true that plant respiration is impotent to make any improvement in the hygienic qualities of the air, it might be pertinently asked, What does the respiration of plants consist of, and what are its effects upon the atmosphere? The fact, as above stated, that plants at night respire in precisely the same manner as animals, is correct, and has long been well understood, but it has not until within comparatively recent times been known that they, at least in the majority of instances, likewise exhibit the same process during the day. Thus the respiratory phenomenon in plants, so far from being antagonistic to that in animals, really takes the same course. This view was first put forward by Mohl, and was subsequently to a great extent confirmed by the experiments of M. Coriander (*Revue Scientifique*, August 1, 1884), and since then has been adopted by all the leading vegetable physiologists. The experiments of M. Coriander are of further interest as showing that the very young portions of the plants and young leaves, owing to their containing a greater proportion of nitrogeneous and correspondingly lesser proportion of carbonaceous matter, exhale more carbon dioxide than the older green tissues. This he explains to his own satisfaction by saying that in the case of the bud and the other very young green organs the carbon dioxide liberated during respiration is not so rapidly reduced by the act of the assimilative function, which, be it remembered, is the exact reverse of the respiratory, as in the more mature organs of the plants in which the hydrocarbons are more rapidly deposited. Now, the explanation of the diurnal respiration of plants having for so long a time escaped observation is to be found in the fact that assimilation is distilling oxygen into the atmosphere with greatly more energy, thus really concealing the feebler process of respiration.

From the foregoing observations upon these two distinct processes carried on by the leaves of plants, it will be at once evident that the effect of the one assimilation upon the respirable medium is decidedly beneficial, purifying it, while that of the other, respiration, is injurious, if it have any effect whatever.

This brings us to the second inquiry respecting the respiratory act in plants, namely, what are the actual sanitary relations of plant-breathing? That illustrious man of science, Professor von Pettenkofer, has, after carefully investigating the question, boldly stated the proposition that none whatever could be proven to exist ("Hygienic Influence of Plants," *loc. cit.*, February, 1878). As has been already remarked, the view quite universally held by hygienists of a single generation ago was that plants, by diffusing carbon dioxide at night, really do vitiate the atmosphere; some of them even going so far as to assert that in a closed apartment, for example, in which shrubs had been imprudently left, the air was as much depraved by them as though it had been occupied by an equal number of persons. Owing to the great practical importance of this question, it is incumbent to sift carefully the evidence at hand tending to maintain the dictum of Professor von Pettenkofer. To fortify his position, Von Pettenkofer first proceeds to show the constancy of the amount of carbon dioxide present in the air, which amount, setting aside severe storms or very thick fog, ranges, as is well known, from three to four parts in each ten thousand of the volume of the air. The proportion of carbon dioxide in apartments occupied by man has been frequently determined, and the quantity is commonly taken as the criterion of the quality of the atmosphere. One per mille is usually regarded as marking the boundary line between good and bad air.

The reader will here be asked to give ear to an account of sundry experiments relating to this essentially important sanitary question, which narrative is based in great part upon Professor von Pettenkofer's own record of data tending to support his proposition, which maintains that the amount of carbon dioxide over larger or smaller areas or tracts of country does not, so far as concerns the influence of vegetation upon this element, exhibit differences to the extent of one per mille.

In 1830, De Saussure began to make researches into the variations in the quality of carbon dioxide in Geneva, and they were about ten years later continued by

Bevoer of Holland and Boussingault in Paris. In more recent times a great number of experiments on the subject by Roscoe in Manchester, Schultz at Rostock, and Pettenkofer and his pupils, particularly Dr. Wolfhugel at Munich, have been recorded. The results show that as the methods of determining facts have been perfected, the variations—very small from the first—have been found to be still smaller. Working by a method liable to give an excess, Saussure found from 3.7 to 6.2 parts in 10,000. According to this experimentalist, there were also observed slight differences between winter and summer, day and night, town and country, land and sea, mountains and valleys, which were ascribed to vegetation. The experiments of Boussingault, however, show the per centum of carbon dioxide to be rather lower, and give about the same mean for Paris and St. Cloud, the former being 4.13 and the latter place 4.14 in 10,000. Having considered that in Paris not less than 2,944,000 litres of carbon dioxide were exhaled by men, animals, and fuel, Boussingault was greatly astonished at this result. At Rostock, Schultz found the atmosphere to contain from 2.5 to 4 parts of carbon dioxide in 10,000. On an average it was somewhat greater when the wind blew off shore than off the sea. Experiments by the celebrated Roscoe have been made on the air at a station in the centre of Manchester and at two stations in the country. To his great astonishment, Roscoe discovered that the air in the space in front of Owen's College contained no more carbon dioxide than the air at the country stations, for he had thought that the vast manufactories of Manchester, in which coal was largely consumed, must exercise a marked effect upon the amount of this substance in the air. The greatest amount present was found during one of the thick fogs which prevail in England. He occasionally observed variations, but, strange as it may seem, when the proportion of carbon dioxide increased or diminished it most generally was exactly the same in the country. The observations of Wolfhugel in Munich showed the carbon to be between 3 and 4 parts in 10,000. It seldom happened that he observed variations, the maximum being 6.9 parts in 10,000 in very thick fog, the minimum 1.5 parts in 10,000 in a heavy snow-storm, when the mercury was very low in the barometer. In this connection the ingenious investigations of Professor Liebig may not prove uninteresting, since they so fully confirm the view of the invariability of the composition of our atmosphere for perhaps untold ages back.

It was the custom of the Roman ladies on the death of persons dear to them to collect their tears in little glass vases, which, after being partly filled, were hermetically sealed and placed in the sarcophagus with the dead. This celebrated chemist took one of these lachrymal vases, broke it, and analyzed its contents, when to his utter amazement he found that the air was of exactly the same composition as the medium which we of the present day respire.

The reader may here be pardoned for desiring to know why the very great quantity of this substance poured into the air in a city like Manchester or Paris fails to raise sensibly the per centum of carbon dioxide.

The answer, as pointed out by Von Pettenkofer ("Hygienic Influence of Plants," *loc. cit.*), is very simple; namely, by rarefaction in the currents of the atmosphere. According to the same observer, we are apt not to take this factor into account, but think rather of the air as stagnant. The average velocity of the air is about three metres per second; hence, assuming a column of air one hundred feet high and of mean velocity, he has reckoned that the carbon dioxide from the lungs and chimneys of Paris or Manchester is not sufficient to increase the amount so that it can be detected by our present methods. Again, in the same conservative spirit, he asks us to consider first the mobility of the air, and then the mass of the air encompassing the earth. The weight of this mass is, as the barometer tells us, equal to that of a layer of mercury which would cover the surface of the earth to the depth of seven hundred and sixty millimetres (more than three-quarters of a metre). From the weight of this, several billion kilometres, some idea can be formed of the volume of the air, and when we consider that air, even beneath a pressure of seven hundred and sixty millimetres of mercury, is yet 10.395 times lighter than mercury, surely, in masses like these, variations such as those spoken of go for nothing. While the fact that the carbon dioxide contained in all vegetable life is absorbed as such and derived chiefly from the atmosphere, though to a slight extent from water and the soil, is incontrovertible, it is equally certain that the air of the green wood contains no less carbon dioxide than the air in the largest city or on an extensive tract of waste land, or, as Von Pettenkofer assures us, that the air in the Sahara so called of Munich, formerly called the Dultplatz, contains no more carbon dioxide than the neighboring Eslchen-ground. The proof of this assertion is indisputable. For him Dr. Nittel brought several specimens of air in hermetically-sealed glass tubes from his travels in the Libyan Desert, from sandy wastes, and from oases on which he could conveniently make experiments at Munich. The results proved the amount of carbon dioxide to be just the same for the greenest oases as for the barren wastes. If it were deemed necessary, not less incontestable proof to show the unchanging character of the quantity of oxygen in the air could be furnished. Upon good authority it may be affirmed that the air on the summit of Mont Blanc has not been found to differ from that of the city or in the swamps of Bengal. Nor is it greater in the sea air or forest than in the air of the most arid desert. Despite, therefore, the well-established facts that plants on the one hand display the function of emitting oxygen under the influence of light, absorbing simultaneously carbon dioxide, and on the other a true respiration consisting in giving off carbon dioxide and withdrawing from the air oxygen, it can certainly be concluded that the effect of these functions upon the composition of the air is absolutely inappreciable.

So stands the case in relation to the action of these two plant functions upon the outer air; but let us next inquire whether or not, when plants are kept in confined spaces, as, *per example*, in living-rooms, the case is not altered. We well know that while the largest concourse of human beings in the open air produces no perceptible effect upon the amount of carbon dioxide in the air, a crowded public hall or closed apartment *in-*

variably shows an increase in the percentage of this substance. It is stated upon good authority that owing to the exhalation of carbon dioxide in human respiration of an ordinary-sized family, and in the burning of coal, gas, etc., this substance is quite generally found in amounts greater than in the open air. Such facts would seem to warrant the expectation of obtaining similar results in a room at night filled with plants and flowers. Again, in the day, when assimilation is actively conducted, should not the air of a room filled with plants show an increase in the per centum of oxygen? Since the science of hygiene has again come to occupy a place in the foremost ranks of medical research, the above questions demand close and dispassionate scrutiny; at all events, to pursue any other course would fail to satisfy the intelligent and thinking masses. In the first place, it has been well argued that the production of matter by plants is a comparatively slow process; thus, matters requiring but a brief period for absorption and subsequent decomposition in the animal whereby as much oxygen has been consumed as was liberated in the production of it, has required an immensely longer period of time for its preparation by the plant. A clear conception of this difference in functional activities between the animal and vegetable organisms can be formed by reflecting for a single moment how slow the process of growth of wheat before it can be eaten as bread, which a man will eat, digest, and decompose in twenty-four hours. Considerations such as these would of themselves seem to render it doubtful whether plants, when kept in closed rooms, would produce enough either of oxygen in the day or carbon dioxide in the night to make any perceptible difference in the quantities of these gaseous bodies. But here the careful experiments of Von Pettenkofer again aid us in arriving at a satisfactory solution of the point under consideration; and it is my purpose to do him the honor to let him tell the story of his labors after his own happy fashion: " It would scarcely be intelligible if I were to calculate how much carbon dioxide a rose, a geranium, or a begonia would absorb and give out in a room in a day, and to what extent the air might be changed by it, taking into account the inevitable change of air always going on. I will draw attention to a concrete case. When the Royal Winter Garden in Munich was completed and in use, it occurred to me to make experiments on the effect of the whole garden on the air within it. There could not be a more favorable opportunity for experimenting on the air in a space full of vegetation. This green and blooming space was not exposed to the free currents of air which at once immensely rarefy all gaseous exhalations, but was kept warm under a dome of glass through which only the light of heaven penetrated. Although not hermetically sealed, the circulation of air in such a building, compared with that in the open air, is reduced over a hundred thousand fold. I asked permission to make experiments for several days, at various hours of the day and night, which was readily granted. Now, what was the result? The proportion of carbonic acid in the Winter Garden was almost as high as in the open air. This greatly surprised me, but I hoped at any rate to have one of my traditional ideas confirmed. I hoped to find less carbonic acid in the day than in the night, supported by the fact that the green portions of plants under the influence of light decomposed carbonic acid and developed oxygen. But even here I was disappointed. I generally found carbonic acid increasing from morning till evening, and decreasing from night till morning. As this seemed really paradoxical, I doubled my tests and care, but the results remained the same. At that time I knew nothing of the large amount of carbonic acid of the air, in the soil, the air of the ground, or I should probably have been less surprised.

" One day it became suddenly clear to me why there was always more carbonic acid by day than by night. I had been thinking only of the turf, the shrubs, and trees which consumed carbonic acid and produced oxygen, and not of the men and birds in the Winter Garden. One day when there were considerably more men at work there than usual, the carbonic acid rose to the highest point, and sank again to the average during the night. The production of carbonic acid by the working and breathing of human beings was so much greater than that consumed by the plants in the same time."

From the nature of the results of his experiments, Professor von Pettenkofer justly concludes that the amount of carbon dioxide in the air in the Winter Garden cannot be reckoned as telling for or against the hygienic value of vegetation in an enclosed space. The above experiments speak for themselves. It is worthy of particular mention, however, that, contrary to the old and widespread traditional notion that plants, by giving out carbonic dioxide at night, render the air harmful, there was found to be even less of this gas present than in the daytime. The explanation of this point is of signal importance. It does not attempt to disprove the power plants have to develop carbon dioxide, but the production of this gas by the working and breathing of human beings in the daytime being so greatly in excess of what the plants give out at night, the latter becomes almost inappreciable. On these grounds there can be, therefore, no valid objection to the practice of keeping plants in living- and sleeping-apartments. As the evidences, the result of scientific research, accumulate, traditional errors must sooner or later vanish. The oxygen in the Winter Garden this illustrious savant found to be rather higher than in the open air; there it was about twenty-one per cent., and in the Winter Garden twenty-two to twenty-three per cent. Let us also inquire into the sanitary value of the slight increase of oxygen observed by this noted investigator. In this connection it is to be remembered that oxygen is absolutely indispensable to maintain both animal and vegetable life; also that the normal proportion of oxygen by bulk in the atmosphere is about one-fifth. Now, the quantity needful for the purposes of the human economy is, practically speaking, constant, the amount present in the air we breathe being, therefore, no criterion of the amount actually consumed by us. Thus, at six thousand feet above the level of the sea, the air with the same temperature is one-fifth rarefied, there being a fifth less oxygen in a given area; hence, to inhale the same amount of oxygen as at sea-level, it is clear that a fifth more atmosphere is needful. To meet this increased task, the respirations are comparatively more rapid and the operations of the circulatory function in like manner.

"When I came to Colorado, seven years ago," writes Dr. Dennison ("Rocky Mountain Health Resorts," p. 82), "I noticed an increase in my respirations from about twenty to thirty in twenty-four hours, while rising four thousand feet in Kansas, and an increase of pulsation from seventy to eighty-two." According to Dr. Vacher, the surviving aeronaut in the Zenith, M. Gasten Tessandier gave him the record of his respirations as twenty-six at seventeen thousand three hundred and thirty-one feet, and on the earth nineteen to twenty-three per minute. When he went to investigate the remarkable effect of the Winter Air Cave (Caves d'Air) at Davos, Dr. Vacher made a careful estimate of his respirations, which were 18.2 per minute ("Le Mont Dores-Davos, Étude Médicale et Climatologique," etc., quoted by Dennison).

Inasmuch as it is clearly established on the one hand that we respire no less oxygen in a rarefied than in air at sea-level, so on the other can it be readily shown that when we breathe an atmosphere containing an excess of oxygen the effect is not to produce a more rapid transformation of matter, or, in other words, to consume a larger amount of oxygen. As in an air of less than average density the number of respirations are increased, so in an atmosphere of greater than normal density the number of inhalations are in a corresponding ratio diminished. Thus, for instance, divers, who breathe highly compressed air very rich in oxygen, find it necessary to respire only about ten times per minute, against a normal average which is seventeen. This view is also fully confirmed by the experiments of Lavoisier, as well as by those of Regnault and Reiset (quoted by Pouchet, *loc. cit.*). These gentlemen placed animals for twenty-four hours in air very rich in oxygen, but they did not consume more of it than in the ordinary air. According to Von Pettenkofer, in the case of healthy individuals neither an increase nor decrease of one or two per cent. of oxygen does harm, for under ordinary circumstances we inhale one-fourth of the oxygen in the air we breathe; we inhale it with twenty-one per cent. and exhale it with sixteen per cent. From all of the above evidence, it is clear that the influence of the slight increase in the proportion of oxygen resulting from the action of plants upon the health of the members of the household is quite inconsiderable. While, therefore, the plant functions which we have considered, namely, assimilation and respiration, exercise no perceptible hygienic influence, the main object of the discussion has been to endeavor to show the utter folly of attributing to these functions hurtful influences.

The absorption of moisture by plants is a physiological process which has in recent times attracted considerable attention, and is one concerning which the opinions of our ablest botanists are singularly at variance. It has been long recognized that the moisture found in plant structures and the currents passing through them are derived chiefly from the soil, and are taken up by the absorbent action of the rootlets. This process on the part of living plants of absorbing water is dependent upon certain conditions which ought to be well understood, but unfortunately space forbids more than an incidental mention of them. The evaporation which in the daytime constantly proceeds from the leaves during fair weather causes a movement of water, taking the form of a current from the roots to the leaves of the plant. The effect of this movement upon the absorbing surfaces of the root is to induce a process of suction. To properly grasp what is meant by the latter term, let the reader take a leafy branch which has just been cut off, place the cut surface in water, and it will imbibe sufficient water for purposes of transpiration, *or* even in some instances to develop and put forth fresh foliage. Another condition entirely independent of the foregoing is caused by the roots, and in botanical works is spoken of as *root-pressure*. But the question which at present writing chiefly concerns us and also has given rise to quite an animated controversy is whether plants, through the stomata in their foliage, abstract moisture from the atmosphere. It is obvious to even a casual observer that if they be capable of discharging this function, plants cultivated within-doors, where the air ordinarily contains too little humidity, would have a more or less deleterious influence.

That plants possess the function in question was the opinion of the ancients, attention having been called to it more particularly by Theophrastus. The French philosopher Mariotte, by the following simple though beautiful experiment, endeavored to demonstrate the absorbing power of the leaves. He took a bifurcated branch and placed one part of it in a vessel filled with water, while the other remained exposed to the air. The water absorbed by the former sufficed to keep the latter green and fresh for a long time. From this he concluded the one absorbed for the other. (Pouchet, *loc. cit.*, p. 28.) It is to be remarked, however, that the portion of the branch employed by Mariotte, placed in the water, was entirely prohibited from performing transpiration, which, as we shall see hereafter, is an extremely active process, and the evaporation from the portion exposed to the air creating, in the manner previously described, suction upon the leaves bathed in the water, naturally constitute two conditions strongly favoring the attainment of Mariotte's supposed demonstration, but which conditions certainly do not obtain in the plant during its normal growth. It has been and perhaps still is the universal opinion among gardeners that living plants have the power to absorb moisture, both in the liquid and gaseous state, through their leaves. This belief accounts for their zeal in the use of water to the foliage of plants, not alone for the purpose of washing off dust and insects, but with a view of supplying water for the purposes of growth.

This view, however, was opposed to the one enjoying the greatest favor for a long time after the experiments of Mariotte among vegetable physiologists, such celebrated investigators as De Candolle, Ducharte, and Sachs having determined to their own satisfaction that under normal conditions plants are not, to any extent at least, capable of taking in moisture through their foliage. Thus the illustrious authority Sachs has stated ("Text-Book of Botany," English ed., p. 613) that, "As long as tissues and leaves of uninjured plants with roots become turgid and are supplied with water from below, very considerable absorption through the surface of the leaves themselves, if they are already quite moist, is not to be expected, and it is not easy to suppose the water can go in cells that are already gorged." As every one knows, a withered plant will, when placed in a moist air or when its leaves are wetted, show signs of almost immediate revival. This fact is by Sachs (*loc. cit.*) explained in the following terms: "When land plants wither on a hot day and revive again in the evening, this is the result of diminished transpiration with the decrease of temperature and an increase of the moisture in the air in the evening, the activity of the roots continuing, and not of any absorption of aqueous vapor or dew through the leaves. Rain again revives withered leaves not by penetrating the leaves, but by moistening them and thus hindering further transpiration, and conveying water to the roots, which they then conduct to the leaves."

According to the same observer (*loc. cit.*, p. 613), a simple experiment will afford much instruction to the inquiring mind relating to the question under discussion. "The pot in which a leafy plant is growing is enclosed in a glass or metal vessel provided above with a lid in two portions, and surrounding the stem so as to cover completely the earth in the pot. If the soil is dry, the plant withers. If a bell-glass is placed over it the plant revives, and again withers if it is removed." This revival he believes to be due to diminished evaporation from the leaves when the roots convey but very little water to the plant, while the withering is caused by the fact that the quantity of water supplied by the roots is inadequate to meet the demands of the process of transpiration in the open air.

In support of this view there are recorded the observations of Ducharte, who found that a number of various species, such as Hortensia, Helianthus annuus; also Tillandsias, epidendral Orchids, etc., did not, after withering in the evening in consequence of the dryness of the earth in the pots, recover or become turgid if copiously moistened by dew during a whole night, the pot in which the roots spread being provided with a closed cover. Again, according to the researches of Unger ("Wilhelm der Baden und der Wald," p. 19, quoted by Marsh), the theory of the absorption of watery vapor by the leaves of growing plants is untenable. The writer's own observations relating to this truly occult function tend to confirm the results attained by the investigations already cited.

A growing pot-plant (geranium) in a thrifty condition was experimented with. The whole of the pot was covered with a double layer of oiled silk and the free portion accurately adjusted around the base of the stem, on which it was tied with elastic cord. Thus prepared, no evaporation could take place from the soil in the pot, and, what is of still greater importance, no moisture excepting that which was contained in the soil in the pot could be supplied to the roots. The plant was then placed under a glass case, which was situated over a shallow box in which there was about four inches of soil, which was kept saturated so that the evaporation from it kept the air of the glass chamber quite moist. The whole arrangement was placed near a window having a southern exposure, the plant in clear weather catching the rays of the sun for about five hours of the day. In this situation the plant remained dormant, so far as any visible growth or development was concerned, for about two weeks, when it began to appear languid and the margins of the leaves to change in color, showing slight signs of failing nutrition. The explanation of this long state of apparent hibernation to the plant is simple. The air in the case being so moist as to allow of little or no transpiration, the plant retained the moisture in the pot for the purposes of nutrition only; and since the plant most probably grew but little during that period, there was sufficient water in the pot for its uses..

At the end of two weeks the plant was taken out of the glass case and placed in a sick-chamber having the same exposure, in which chamber three dozen other thrifty plants were growing. The oil silk was allowed to remain, and no water was supplied to the roots. The atmosphere of the room, though agreeable, was noticeably moist to the senses. Here the sun's rays had an opportunity of exciting the plant to transpire actively, and consequently in a few days nutritive changes became very decided, leaf after leaf dying, until at the end of another fortnight a few much-withered leaves only remained. Now, although the methods employed in this experiment may not have given results sufficiently conclusive to assure us that absorption of moisture by the leaves is impossible, they appeared to show that not sufficient aqueous vapor was taken in through the aerial organs to carry on the natural functions of the plant, and not only so, but they seemed to render it highly probable that the chief if not the only source of moisture to the growing plant was through the roots ("Forests, their Influence upon Climate and Rain-fall," by the author).

Whilst we have adduced considerable evidence bearing the stamp of scientific accuracy to disprove the ancient theory which regards the leaves of plants as agents of absorption, it is also to be noted that there have been, and more especially in recent times, recorded by various observers numerous experiments going far towards establishing a contrary view. Upon this point there is quite valuable and conclusive evidence. A number of experiments conducted by Boussingault showed that plants growing in humid atmosphere could absorb moisture only when they had previously lost a portion of their water of constitution,—*i.e.*, that which is essential to their normal existence. Thus, a wilted branch of periwinkle weighing only 4 grammes, after remaining for a day and a half in an atmosphere saturated with aqueous vapor, weighed 4.2 grammes; after twelve hours' immersion in water it weighed 9.4 grammes. The results of the interesting experiments of Rev. George Winslow appeared to be in perfect accord with those of the French savant. Among others, the two following observations by Winslow are in this connection of signal importance. A long series of cut leaves and slips were gathered at 4 P.M., then exposed to sun and wind for three hours, then carefully weighed and exposed all night to dew. At 7.30 A.M., after having been dried, they were again weighed, and all had gained weight and quite recovered their freshness, proving that slightly wetted detached portions do absorb dew.

In the next place, plants growing in pots and of which the earth was not watered were kept alive by the ends of one or more roots being placed in water;

e.g., Mimulus moschatus not only grew vigorously and developed, but also blossomed. Applying the results of his experiments, Mr. Winslow also presents some valuable hints regarding the best mode of preparing and preserving bouquets of cut flowers. "If some plants have buds upon them, let the stalks long, and allow a few leaves to remain on and be also immersed in water, and the buds will then be often found to expand successively. The cut end, to be more absorbed than it otherwise would be, should be again cut off under water. If the blossoms be on a ligneous stem, as of lilac, then the loss of water by evaporation is greater than the woody stalk can supply, so that in this case the addition of leaves in the water will greatly aid, and retain the bunch of flowers fresh for a long time. On the other hand, if a blossom be already about to shed its petals, then the additional supply of water furnished by the leaves on the stalk appears to hasten the coming dissolution, and the flower perishes rather sooner than it would otherwise do. The water must be changed every day and the submerged leaves must be lightly wiped with a cloth, as by endosmotic action they soon become more or less coated with mucus. No leaves must be in water unless perfectly green and of vigorous growth" (see article on the absorption of water by leaves of plants, A. W. Bennet, *American Naturalist*, vol. xiii. p. 20).

With the results of the experiments by Winslow, those of Cailletet relative to the same subject are in the main concordant. His results seem equally worthy to be briefly enumerated. They successfully demonstrate the useful fact that a plant growing in a humid soil and receiving by its roots the quantity of water necessary to its normal condition does not absorb the water which moistens its leaves, but such absorption takes place as soon as the leaves begin to wither, in consequence of the desiccation of the soil. In this way is to be explained the phenomenon of certain plants maintaining a healthy condition without any contact with the soil and even absolutely isolated from all assimilable substances. Thus, specimens of Pourretea, a rootless, bromeliaceous plant, maintained a healthy existence and exhibited considerable increase in weight while suspended for more than six years in the air by a wire. No moisture except that from the gardener's syringe ever reached it, and yet it was continually putting out new leaves and abundantly flowering (*Gardener's Monthly*, February, 1873). The mode of living in this case exhibited by the Pourretea precisely answers to that displayed by so-called air-plants, known to the scientific botanist as epiphytes, which have connection neither with the soil nor the juices of the other plants upon which they prey, but imbibe directly all the moisture they require from the air. It should be here noted that with regard to plants living in a manner purely predaceous the case is quite different, since the terminal rootlets of the latter dip into the juices of their host and absorb from them the needful amount of nutriment for their sustenance.

From the proof brought forward tending both to confirm and to refute the theory of the absorption of moisture by plant foliage, it will appear obvious that the question is one respecting which there is great division of opinion, and hence we may not as yet be in a position to render an absolute decision. It may, however, be gravely affirmed that the balance of argument, more particularly the results of the skilled labors of the more modern works in this field of research, seems to be in favor of the view that plants possess the function in question; it must, however, be distinctly understood to hold only when they are placed in unfavorable circumstances for absorption by their roots.

Two inferences appear to be pretty clearly established by the numerous skilful experiments above detailed. The one which is to be drawn from the labors of the opponents of the theory may be stated as follows: that growing, including potted plants, when well watered and liberally supplied with the proper soil, imbibe, practically speaking, no aqueous vapor from the air. The other which is to be drawn from the experimental results of those endeavoring to carry the theory to an actual demonstration may be formulated thus: that all plants which do not receive sufficient water from the earth in which their roots are imbedded to keep them in vigorous growth, or, in other words, if plants be allowed to wither, can by virtue of the power the leaves possess to take on vicarious absorptive actions recover their natural freshness. In view of such facts, the old idea which has been and in some quarters still is held, namely, that plants growing in a properly moistened soil also obtain a certain share of moisture directly from the air, is doubtless illusory. On the other hand, the field botanist who sprinkles the plants in his vasculum in order to keep them alive and green till he reaches home is acting in harmony with an established physiological law. We cannot, after again overlooking the deductions made from all the experimental data at hand relating to the question of absorption of moisture by the foliar organs of the plant, find any ground of objection against the practice of keeping plants in living-apartments, provided the earth in which they grow is kept sufficiently moist to supply all the demands of nutrition. As we shall see hereafter, the rate at which living plants emit aqueous vapor from their leaves is so vastly in excess of the possible limit of absorption that the effects of the latter are really inappreciable, and, furthermore, it will appear clear that instead of diminishing they largely increase the atmospheric humidity. The subject of leaf-absorption having engaged the attention of numerous vegetable physiologists, and being one of great practical moment as well as philosophic interest, it has been deemed desirable to give a rather full exposition of the different views advanced by those who at different times made it an experimental study.

CHAPTER III.

House-plants and malaria—Brief description of malaria—Intermittent and remittent types—Dumb ague—The cause a specific ferment—Is not the result of organic decomposition—The conditions essential to the production of malaria—The possibility of house-plants causing malaria, and how this can be averted—The victims of malaria—Effect of odorous emanations—Most of them delightful—A few of them only are injurious—The scent of roses—Objections to living plants within dwellings answered.

THE famous bacteriologist Professor Tommasi Crudeli has recently directed attention to the newly discovered and practical fact that house-plants have been known to produce symptoms of malaria.

Now, although this novel idea, which assumes to endow growing plants with the power to generate a much-dreaded affection, can be readily shown to be opposed to all traditional views upon the subject, nevertheless, emanating as it does from one eminent for medical learning and at the same time an exceedingly zealous original investigator, it surely is entitled to most respectful consideration.

Before entering into a discussion of this point, however, it is my purpose to proceed to a brief consideration of the subject of malaria in general, and to examine into its causative relations in particular; believing that such a course will greatly aid the reader in reaching a wise and safe decision of the question raised by this noted Italian observer.

Moreover, if the readers deem it necessary to offer

additional reasons for pursuing this method, we would simply ask them to note the ever-increasing popular interest, which may be largely owing to the increasing prevalence of the disease, everywhere shown in the subject of malaria. Its baneful effects seem to-day to be almost universally recognized and in no small degree appreciated. Thus, to show the great importance which popularly attaches to the phenomena exhibited by this disease, it need only be observed that in the selection of a permanent home a locality found by experience to be highly malarious is, without regard to any superior advantages it may possess, prudently condemned.

Prior to the introduction of the term malaria, this affection had been known chiefly as marsh miasm, a phrase introduced in 1717 by the Italian writer Lancisci; this name being applied to it because of the fact that it had been supposed to be solely attributable to vegetable decomposition in marshy localities. As will appear hereafter, this doctrine, in the light of later observations, lacks full confirmation. On account of the term marsh miasm or paludal fever being too restricted in its application, another author, McCulloch, in 1827, introduced into English literature the term malaria, which possesses the advantage of being more comprehensive, including as it does the well-known intermittent and remittent forms of fever as well as so-called "dumb ague." Among the inhabitants of Italy the term malaria had been colloquial, and in our own country it has from the time of its first employment to designate the disease in question been very generally adopted, not only by the medical profession but also by the laity. The disease is also popularly known by such various titles as "chills and fever," "the shakes," "fever and ague," "fever of the country," and so on. It does not seem incumbent to describe at length the symtomatology as expressed in the varied types of the affection; besides, this aspect of the case is one which does not at present writing so much concern us, but to portray the disease in mere outline may, it is hoped, be incidentally useful if not absolutely essential. The onset of an attack of intermittent fever or ague is in nearly all instances characterized by marked chills, usually accompanied by more or less tremor of the muscular system, and more particularly the muscles of the lower jaw, to the extent, in most cases, of causing "chattering of the teeth." This stage lasts all the way from a few minutes to two hours, and is immediately followed by a stage of fever, in which there is a notable elevation of temperature, the skin at the same time remaining hot and dry. The second is longer than the first stage, varying from three to eight hours, and terminates in the third or sweating stage, which closes the scene attending one paroxysm. Then follows an intermission of one, two, three, or more days, during which interval there is an entire absence of fever, probably to be succeeded by a recurring "shaker." Of this form of fever there are three types, each having a definite interval, or in other words each variety manifesting in the return of the paroxysms a distinct law of periodicity. Thus we have the quotidian, in which the paroxysms occur at intervals of twenty-four hours, the tertian, at intervals of forty-eight hours, while in the quartan type this period is seventy-two hours. The remittent is less frequently met with than the intermittent form of malarial fever. This is true at least of temperate climes. The best authorities look upon it as a modification of intermittent fever, severer in type, however, and frequently demanding not a little diagnostic skill on the part of the clinician to distinguish it from certain other affections. Hence to do full justice to the subject would not only consume too much space, but also fail to be either interesting or profitable to the general reader. The ill-defined and variable symptoms presented by "dumb ague" form an interesting type for the student of disease-phenomena. Though greatly diversified as to its manifestations, there can be no doubt that persons who are more or less indisposed frequently have a feeling of confidence that they are suffering from some form of malaria when in truth they are affected with some other disorder having symptoms almost identical. In the experience of the busy practitioner, more particularly if he resides in a malarious locality, it is not an unusual occurrence for patients to present themselves for treatment and forestall his own opinion by stating without hesitation that they are suffering from malaria, though the physician, after making careful examination of their condition, is obliged to give an opinion at variance with their prepossessions, the real difficulty being found to be simply an ordinary cold, or a condition known as biliousness or other complaint. A practical lesson of no mean importance to be drawn from all this might profitably be formulated thus: Do not be too ready to believe you are suffering from malarial poisoning unless you, at some previous time, have had the disease, or it has taken an unmistakable form in which severe chills have been followed by fever and this in turn by profuse sweating, and these periodical exacerbations have been and still are occurring at regular intervals; but seek the advice of your trusted physician, making sure at the same time that he is not a mere pretentious charlatan. The following are perhaps the symptoms which most nearly determine what are commonly regarded as latent forms of malaria, and they are added to the above detailed account of the disease with a view simply to assist those who enlist in the noble and refining practice of cultivating plants in their dwellings in deciding whether any manifestations of illness developing in themselves are, in point of fact, symptoms of malaria or those of one of the many closely-allied disorders arising from other causes. It is to be particularly noted that any one of the three stages already described as constituting a fit of intermittent fever may be entirely wanting, while the remaining two may be but feebly expressed. Upon close observation there will usually be found to be an irregular, or rarely a regular periodicity about the attack. While serving in the capacity of resident physician of the Episcopal Hospital at Philadelphia, and subsequently in that of visiting physician to the out-patient department of the same institution, where numerous patients suffering from the various forms of this dread affection are daily prescribed for, there has been offered an exceptionally good opportunity to verify the observation that those applying for relief from this disease have, upon being questioned, in most cases, assented to having alternately their "good" and their "bad days." The functional activity of the liver is in these subjects greatly impaired, as evidenced by headache and undue drowsiness; upon the tongue is found a thin white coating, which in quite a large proportion of instances has, according to my own observation, a somewhat bluish tint. In his excellent treatise on "The Principles and Practice of Medicine," the late Professor Austin Flint has with commendable insight recommended the use of the clinical thermometer, by means of which any "periodical rise of temperature, when the surface of the body may not show an increase of heat and the pulse is but little accelerated," may be detected. The free use of quinia, which in cases of malaria operates as a specific agent, also serves to aid to complete the diagnosis of cases that would otherwise remain suspicious, or in other words could not be definitely settled by the best diagnostic skill of the physician. It is earnestly hoped that a sufficiently full description of the disease has now been given to render it unnecessary to urge a prudent caution against the too general fashion of indiscriminately pronouncing any given case of illness to be malaria and at once attempting to find an explanation of its appearance.

Than the subject of the true nature of the causes of malaria and the various conditions under which they become operative, none of greater importance or interest could be presented. From the time of the introduction of the term marsh miasm by Lancisci in the beginning of the eighteenth century down to within recent years, the doctrine that the morbific agent was the result of vegetable decomposition in marshy districts held universal sway. That the majority of marshy localities are malarious is undeniable. There is, however, a notable exception in the case of salt-water marshes, which places, strange as it may seem to the practically-minded, non-professional reader, enjoy almost perfect freedom from the disease. It is, moreover, to be remarked that by mixing salt and fresh water, as happens in certain marshes in the State of New Jersey and in the many swamps of the West Indies, we have conditions which in a striking degree favor the development of malaria. The particular localities where the ravages of the disease most extensively predominate are the deltas and estuaries of rivers, as well as smaller streams, which are apt to be inundated. Among familiar though striking examples are the Ganges, Euphrates, and the Mississippi Rivers. To place beyond doubt the falsity of the old hypothesis which gravely assumed the disease to be caused only by the emanations arising from organic decomposition in marshy localities, it is simply necessary to direct attention to the fact that the disease not infrequently occurs in places where the conditions are almost directly opposed. Thus we may mention "barren rocks" (Ionian Islands, Hong-Kong, parts of Beloochistan, De Los Islands near Sierra Leone); high table-lands more or less barren (Deccan, Mysore, Persia, New Castile); mountainous regions (Andes, Rocky Mountains, prairies of North America, and savannas of Venezuela and Brazil) (Encyclopedia Britannica). After making a series of delicate experiments upon aquatic algæ obtained from malarious localities, Salisbury, in the month of January, 1866 (see

American Journal of the Medical Sciences), announced to the medical profession the discovery of the Palmella gemiasma, which he held to be the specific agent in the production of malaria. About the same time still other observers of note were zealously applying themselves to the investigations of these low forms of vegetable life, and although each savant had, as the result of his skilful labors, been successful in demonstrating to his own satisfaction the causative agent of malaria, strangely enough each had pointed out a different variety of alga. It also was subsequently found that in not a single instance had these results been carried to a successful demonstration, and it is to be particularly noted that the palmella or ague-plant of Salisbury has been found to be absent in many malarious regions, while, on the contrary, it has been found to be present in many places wholly free from malaria. Although down to the year 1879 the hypothetical germ causing malaria had not been discovered, there now appeared on the scene two zealous and already illustrious workers in the field of bacteriology, namely, Klebs and Tommasi Crudeli. As the result of their joint labors, extending over a considerable period of time, these gentlemen have isolated a low vegetable organism, and named it *Bacillus malariæ*, which they claim to be the special agent producing all forms of malaria. Whilst the evidence afforded by the subsequent experiments of these and other observers greatly strengthened the proposition that we have, in this disease, to deal with a schizomycete, yet it is but just to state that certain observations still more recently made in Rome indicate with equal show of reason that the schizomycete of malaria does not at all times assume the exact bacillary form described by Klebs and Tommasi Crudeli. Meanwhile, the point of paramount importance and chief interest to the hygienist has been practically settled, namely, that he has to do with a living ferment. Pertaining to the disease in question there are many familiar facts which can, according to this view, be readily explained. It enables us to comprehend clearly why the malarial poison can flourish in soils of most various chemical composition; why the disease is more prevalent during the warm season, and as a rule in marshy than in non-marshy localities; why it rarely happens that certain marshes with their stagnant waters are exempt, and so on. In an address delivered before the eighth session of the Industrial Congress, Copenhagen, August 12, 1884, and published in the *New York Medical Record*, August 23, 1884, Professor Tommasi Crudeli has, in a highly lucid and practical manner, discussed this curious little living ferment. He has pointed out the conditions favorable to the multiplication of the malarial ferment contained in the soil and to its dispersion through the superjacent atmosphere, inviting attention to three conditions which are absolutely essential, and the concurrence of which is indispensable to the production of malaria. First, a temperature which does not fall below 20 degrees Cent. (67.5 degrees Fahr.); secondly, a very moderate degree of humidity; thirdly, the direct action of the oxygen of the air upon the strata of earth which contain the ferment. If a single one of these three conditions be wanting, the development of malaria becomes impossible. He further calls attention to the fact that not all earth containing this ferment is capable of poisoning the superjacent atmosphere. It is a matter of some practical moment that this germ may, after having lain dormant for an indefinite time, again become active in producing malaria, as, for example, when placed under conditions most favorable for its development and multiplication. Closely associated with this there is another well-known fact, namely, the overturning of a malarial soil whether by means of the plough or the spade, as well as that resulting from the construction of railways, is almost invariably attended by increased prevalence of the disease. To this idea popular experience lends universal support. The explanation is not difficult, and should be properly understood. It will appear obvious that by upturning the soil the surface which is constantly exposed containing this specific ferment is increased, thus giving the essential conditions already described every opportunity of asserting their respective influences to the end of generating malarial miasm. In the article of Professor Crudeli before cited (*loc. cit.*), he has, happily for our further purpose, indicated certain natural and artificial modes of rendering salubrious malarious localities. It sometimes happens that as a result of continuous warm dry weather all the moisture is evaporated from the malarious soil, and it in consequence ceases to generate the disease-producing germ. Likewise does nature rarely obtain the same end by covering a malarious soil with earth which does not contain the malarial ferment, or with a matting formed of earth and the roots of grasses closely growing together in a natural meadow.

Among the various devices which we owe to the

ingenuity of man, there is perhaps none to which attaches more importance than that of drainage. It is regrettable that the subject cannot here be more fully discussed. On account of the extreme activity of the transpiratory function exhibited by growing vegetation and the consequent absorption of the excessive moisture from the soil, it has been recommended to plant trees in marshy localities, and in this way it has been supposed trees might render salubrious a locality more or less malarious. But since the question whether trees are really capable of exercising this happy influence can have no possible bearing upon the subject of the relation of house-plants to malaria, its further discussion will be resumed where it more properly belongs, in a future chapter. Assuming the cause of malaria to be a living ferment, and also the scientific data brought forward by Professor Crudeli to be ample to fully prove this postulate, let us now inquire how plants in living-chambers might generate and multiply the specific germ so as to produce malaria in the inmates, this, the reader will remember, being claimed by the same celebrated authority. To support his own hypothesis Tommasi Crudeli furnishes the following practical record, which, however, was communicated to him by Professor von Eichwald, of St. Petersburg. A Russian lady, who usually enjoyed good health and who lives in a perfectly salubrious locality, was attacked by an intermittent fever of a true malarial character. The febrile attacks yielded easily to moderate doses of quinia, but a relapse invariably took place when the invalid returned to her ordinary habits of life. The alternations of easy cure and obstinate relapses continued for many months, during which time Professor von Eichwald was unable to discover the cause of this singular affection. One day he was struck by this circumstance: the cure of the attacks was maintained as long as the invalid remained in the bedroom, while the relapse took place when she left that room, even when she did not leave the house. Now, this lady when not suffering passed the greater part of the time in a well-heated drawing-room, containing a considerable number of flower-pots. Professor von Eichwald had them all removed, and from that day the cure was assured and no more relapses occurred. (See also *Am. Jour. Med. Sciences*, January, 1882.) Now, according to the views entertained by Professor Crudeli himself, the malarial germ must remain innocuous excepting when, as before mentioned, three essential conditions are present. To the intelligent observer it will appear obvious that since the temperature of the living-apartments should, according to the teachings of hygienists, range from sixty-five to seventy degrees Fahr., one at least of the indispensable conditions must under these circumstances almost constantly obtain not only during the winter season, when artificial heat is required, but also during the other seasons. It will appear not less clear that the second requirement, which demands a permanent state of humidity of soil, would, if the plants be sufficiently watered, not infrequently prevail. Certain it is that the plants in order to maintain their healthy growth must receive a constant supply of water to their roots. But regarding this question of the connection between the moisture of the soil and the origin of malaria, the best sentiment of the hygienists of the present who have given it serious attention is, while a moist soil eminently favors the development of the specific agent causing malarial affection, an equally potent factor to the same end is a soil either too moist or too dry, or, in other words, a rapid rise or fall of the ground-water is often in great measure responsible for an outbreak of one form among others of this class of diseases. Irregular or excessive watering of plants with pots which do not admit of drainage at the base, therefore, might tend strongly to establish the conditions favorable to the prevalence of paroxysmal fever, and such careless handling of house-plants should scrupulously be avoided by those wishing to introduce them into their homes. Neither would there be the slightest obstacle in the way of the third or remaining essential condition coming into play, since nothing could interfere with the action of the oxygen of the air upon any germs present in the superficial soil of the flower-pots. But the evident fact must be kept in remembrance that while the conditions favorable to the development and multiplication of the malarial germ may at times prevail in our dwellings, they cannot occasion the disease without the existence of the paramount condition, namely, its presence in the soil of the pots in which the plants are growing.

And to every fair-minded person it must be clear that there is available an efficient and easily applicable remedy; for accepting, as we have done, Professor Crudeli's theory of the etiology of malaria, nothing could be more simple than to replace the malarial soil of the flower-pots with non-malarial, or it might be amply sufficient simply to remove the superficial portion of the soil and to cover the remainder in the pot with soil containing no malarial germs. The latter point is one which our gardeners and florists would do well to consider. The importance of ascertaining in the most careful manner whether any given case of malaria occurring in a household in which plants are cultivated is really due to the latter or to some adequate concurrent cause, cannot too strongly be emphasized. Moreover, though contrary to the teachings of Professor Crudeli, it remains to be said that as the result of numerous inquiries from many of the leading practical florists and gardeners of Philadelphia, the disease in not a single instance was found to be ascribable to the influence of the treasures of the greenhouse; and surely no one, except he be unreasonably prejudiced, can for a moment doubt that if plants and flowers do possess the power to generate sufficient of the specific germs to produce malaria, then the practical cultivators of plants who are their constant companions could hardly be so fortunate as to escape the disease. Surely, until more extended reliable observations from the side of clinical experience are reported tending to establish the scientific accuracy of Professor Crudeli's demonstration, more than ordinary precaution is deemed unnecessary.

From the evidence brought to light in this discussion we learn two lessons of no minor consequence. First, that though cases of malaria ascribable to the effects of potted plants will be found to be extremely rare, the possibility of their occurrence should be kept in remembrance. Secondly, in view of the convenience of application and the infallibility of the means at our command to remove the cause whenever found to exist, the folly of discarding plants from living-apartments on the ground of generating malaria will on all hands be readily conceded.

It in all justice remains to be said, however, that to reflect upon having directed attention to the possibility of this new-discovered source of malaria, as well as having pointed out a complete safeguard wherever the proper precautions are vigorously enforced, should bring to the mind of Professor Crudeli great pleasure and satisfaction.

The effects of the odorous emanations from growing plants and beautiful flowers forms an interesting theme for investigation, and is one that has, up to within very recent times, received but little attention. As bearing upon the subject there have been quite recently established certain new facts which have invested the subject with rare interest, but these more important phases, chiefly relating to the power of odorous plants to generate ozone, and the high value accorded to this substance by the sanitarian, will in a future chapter be fully considered. The discussion will be here limited to a consideration of their general, and more particularly their supposed injurious, effects. The great variety of emanations given off by plant life may be merely alluded to as a matter of passing interest. It is to be noted at the outset that the vast majority of them are delightful to the smell, whilst a small proportion only are repugnant or harmful. By the grateful impression they make upon our sense of smell, the fragrant odors emitted from plants are perhaps to most persons little less attractive than the beautiful forms and exquisite colors they present to the sense of sight. In this we discern the beneficent hand of Providence, through vegetable forms which secrete perfumed nectar, ministering to our pleasure and comfort. Though not of any practical moment, it may prove to be incidentally interesting to briefly advert to the industry of collecting and dispensing the various perfumes for toilet purposes. We are told by Homer that men in his day were already familiar with an "oil of roses" and its preparation, and there is no lack of reliable testimony to establish the fact that roses from a remote period of time were cultivated with a view to extracting from them their fragrant essence. It is historically recorded that those illustrious authorities of their day, Galen and Hippocrates, were acquainted with the same product, and, besides using it as a perfume, frequently employed it as a remedial agent. It is stated upon good authority that great quantities of flowers, chief among which is the lavender, grown in the south of France, are used by the London perfumers, the flower season being as anxiously watched there as the grain harvest in other regions. As before intimated, the proportion of odoriferous flowers which are actually productive of baneful effects is quite small, and although it has upon good authority been affirmed that all injurious odors are repulsive, it is erroneous to suppose, as some have done, that all the disagreeable odors exhaled by plants are injurious in their effects upon health. Thus, there is a class of plants whose odors closely resemble those produced by certain animals, Satyrium hircinum (Linn.), for example, which emits a goat-like stench; others emit odors like that of putrid animal flesh, for the express object of alluring certain insects whom they ingeniously deceive into captivity, and, having accomplished their nefarious object, reward them by destroying their existence. As examples of such deliberately deceptive blossoms we may cite the huge parasite discovered by Sir Stamford Raffles in Sumatra, and called for its discoverer *Rafflesia*. This plant has, from the time of its first description, attracted a great deal of attention on all sides, so that a knowledge of its felonious habits has already become familiar even to amateur scientists. But still more curious as well as atrociously wicked are the habits of the wild Arum, or cuckoo-pint. Although not strictly within our province, the story as told by Professor Grant Allen (*Popular Science Monthly*, December, 1884) of the cruel habits of the Arum, which sets up a sort of fly-cage, presents features of sufficient importance and scientific interest to be entitled to a place here, even though it be at the risk of straining the reader's credulity. " This familiar big spring flower exhales a disagreeable, fleshy odor, which by its meat-like flavor attracts a tiny midge, with beautiful iridescent wings and a very poetical name, Psycoda. As in most cases where flies are specially invited, the color of the cuckoo-pint is usually a dull and somewhat livid purple. A palisade of hairs closes the neck of the funnel-shaped blossom, and repeats the lobster-pot tactics of the entirely unconnected South European birthwort. The little flies entering by this narrow and stockaded door, fertilize the future red berries with pollen brought from their last prison, and are then rewarded for their pains by a tiny drop of honey, which slowly oozes from the middle of each embryo fruitlet as soon as it is duly impregnated. Afterwards, the pollen is shed upon their backs by the bursting of the pollen-bags; the hairs wither up, and open the previously barricaded exit, and the midges issue forth in search of a new prison and a second drop of honey.

"This is all strange enough; but stranger still, I strongly suspect the Arum of deliberately hocusing its nectar. I have often seen dozens of these tiny flies roll together in an advanced stage of apparent intoxication upon the pollen-covered floor of an arum-chamber; and the evidences of drunkenness are so clear and numerous that I incline to believe the plant actually makes them drunk in order to insure their staggering about in the pollen and carrying a good supply of it to the next blossom visited."

Whilst the cases cited afford striking illustrations of the great energy with which some plants exhale unpleasant odors, there are others of quite modest appearance, such as wintergreen, rosemint, rosemary, etc., which plants, unlike the former, are with equal activity distilling pleasant aromas into the surrounding medium for a considerable distance. The eminent authority, Pouchet (*loc. cit.*), cites Bartholin, who tells us that the odor of rosemary indicates the coast of Spain more than ten leagues out at sea, and the old historian Diodorus Siculus relates something analogous with respect to Arabia. Some curious instances, many of which are doubtless apocryphal, of the poisonous effects of strong plant-odors, are historically related. Thus, it is held by Pouchet ("The Universe," p. 348) that in the year A.D. 1779 a woman actually died in

London from having kept a large bouquet of irises in her room during the night. According to Preller, a young girl perished in the same way from the effects of a bouquet of violets; and it is recorded that workmen who have imprudently fallen asleep upon bales of saffron have died in consequence. Serious phenomena, writes Pouchet, have been particularly observed in persons keeping nosegays near them during the night. The historian Cramer has briefly related the following cases in point, viz., the death of one of the daughters of Nicholas I., court of Saline (in the department of Jura), and that of a bishop of Poland were attributed to the emanations from roses.

The same authority (*loc. cit.*) gives a few interesting instances in which the scent of roses has been particularly charged with operating deleteriously upon some persons. He writes, Catherine of Thudici could not endure it, and her aversion to flowers was so great that it was enough for her to see a painting of one to be seized with some degree of nausea. The Chevalier de Guise was still more easily affected, for he fainted at the sight of a bunch of roses. To successfully confirm the above with well-authenticated cases of more recent date would, we opine, be impossible; at all events, so far as our examination of the medical literature bearing upon the subject has gone, nothing of the kind has been encountered. In all instances, therefore, in which as the result of floral emanations really dangerous symptoms have been superinduced, a well-marked idiosyncrasy would doubtless have been found to exist. In confirmation of this view it should be stated that Orfila long ago contended that these remarkably odorous exhalations operate like certain poisons, which, while not affecting most persons, act fatally upon certain others. It is, however, undeniable that certain highly-scented flowers, the tuberose and certain lilies, for example, have been known to produce temporary ill effects in the form of various disagreeable symptoms, among them headache, nausea, and faintness being worthy of chief mention. Among the points elsewhere recorded (see "Hygienic and Therapeutic Relations of House-Plants," *Medical Times*, February 6, 1880, p. 15) to be noted in the selection of plants and flowers for in-door cultivation, the following one occurs: those which are highly scented (as the tuberose) should be avoided, because they often give rise to headache and other unpleasant symptoms. The observation, it would appear, has, as the result of ample experience, been pretty well established that the scent of roses, while greatly sought for everywhere, is to some persons very disagreeable and to others very rarely hurtful. Though the subject merits attentive studying, our knowledge of the physiological effects of plant exhalations is unfortunately very limited. To clearly define our views upon this question it will be pardonable to recapitulate a few natural inferences carefully drawn from the facts previously adduced. First, the lethal effects ascribed to plant-odors by some of the ancient writers must be absolutely apocryphal. Secondly, highly-scented flowers, as the tuberose, magnolia glauca, and certain lilies, have an injurious effect, and should in all cases be discarded, so also all plants having intensely disagreeable odors. Thirdly, those emitting milder odors,—the rose, heliotrope, mignonette, for instance,—which flowers occasionally produce unpleasant effects, should whenever found to do so be excluded, but such are not to be totally condemned, since, as will be seen hereafter, the hygienic advantages attendant upon their presence are actually noteworthy. Although at first sight these conclusions may seem somewhat at variance with preceding remarks upon the same subject, it is believed a little serious reflection on the part of the reader will render it clear that they were confined to scrupulously accurate statements of fact.

The various elements tending to show that growing plants and flowers have when cultivated within-doors an injurious influence upon human health, have been now successively discussed, and the only arguments, it will be recollected, having weight worth considering were two in number, namely, that plants under certain conditions seem to be capable of generating malaria, and that they rarely emit odors which exercise a deleterious influence. But we gravely assume that no important evidence has been wanting to show that they really constitute but slight objections, and, what is of greatest importance, we have indicated (*supra*) convenient and efficient safeguards against positive harm from the causes enumerated.

CHAPTER IV.

Hygienic influences of house-plants—Transpiration—Experiments showing its rate, etc.—Effect of transpiration on the dew-point—Table of results—Summary of investigations—Effect of anatomical formation of leaves upon the rate of transpiration—The solar rays the chief exciting cause—Other modifying influences—Obvious effect of transpiration to increase the proportion of moisture in closed rooms—Experiments at the Episcopal Hospital, Philadelphia—Their results proving the ability of plants to increase the degree of humidity of living-rooms—The air of living-rooms also shown to be dryer than the outer air, especially when heated by the hot-air furnace—The effects of transpiration in lowering the temperature—The quantity of atmospheric moisture essential to health—The effect of temperature and relative humidity upon the rate of evaporation from our bodies—Small fluctuations in temperature and degree of saturation of vital moment to preserve health—Moisture furnished by plants highly serviceable where dry furnace heat is employed—The evil effects of furnace heat pointed out—Its relation to bodily ills—Plants becoming the means of obviating distressing symptoms—The high rank taken by plants and flowers as sanitary agencies.

THAT neither sacred nor profane literature prior to the last decade presents anything favoring the idea of vegetable life exercising any valuable hygienic influences, has in the preceding chapters been abundantly verified. On the other hand we are, owing to some recent advances in plant physiology, now enabled happily to show that to growing plants, more particularly when cultivated within dwellings, must be accorded high praise for their actual worth as sanitary agencies. Having made this widely applicable proposition, a study of the various beneficial influences plants and flowers are capable of exerting upon the salubrity of the surrounding air will next engage our earnest attention. There is justification for making this claim for plants chiefly on account of two functions. First, transpiration, or the exhalation of watery vapor from all green portions, but more especially from the green leaves; and, secondly, the generation of ozone by the flower and odoriferous foliage. Their well-known æsthetic influences will also be discussed. Preliminary to making a practical application of our present knowledge of the functions referred to, it is necessary to devote small space to some general considerations, and to carefully examine the experimental studies which have been made thereon, in order that the arguments and conclusions pertaining to the practical issues of our subject may be seen to rest upon the indestructible basis of exact scientific data.

Of the various elements entering into the living portions of plants, water makes up the predominating proportion. The most essential constituent of the living parts of plants, however, is protoplasm, so termed by its discoverer, Dr. Hugo von Mohl. This substance has been defined as that which is sensitive, which moves, appropriates food, and increases in size (Bessey). Its consistence is neither distinctly solid nor liquid, but might be termed semi-fluid or semi-solid, and in the higher orders of plants occupies the cavities, being variously arranged with reference to the vegetable cell-wall. The vegetable, it should be noted, as to its chemical composition and physical properties is identical with animal protoplasm, which unceasingly courses through our veins and nourishes our bodies. The greater the vital activity of this life-giving principle, the more watery is its composition. This is a fact of paramount importance, since it not only serves to show how necessary is water to all the nutritive changes taking place in plants, but also to indicate the power protoplasm possesses to imbibe moisture. Such being the fact, it can be seen that a current is, during the growth of the plant, established from the chief source of all moisture —the soil—in the direction of the more rapidly growing parts, where it is utilized, which current, be it remembered, is to be distinguished from another coursing from the roots to the leaves of the plants for purposes of transpiration. The latter phenomenon may be defined as a natural vaporization of the liquid of the plant, taking place solely from the external surfaces of the living cells, which "on their part remove the water by imbibition from the cell sap."

It is a physiological fact of no little interest that, as Sachs has experimentally shown, the movement of water upward through the stem to supply that which is lost by evaporation occurs solely through the woody tissue or walls of the cells, and not through their cavities, which even in summer, when transpiration is most active, are chiefly filled with air. The true explanation of this phenomenon may with justice be briefly argued to be due to an attraction of the cell-wall for water. This same celebrated authority, it is of further interest to note, has calculated the rapidity of the ascending current of water in a branch of the silver poplar, in which there was strong transpiration, and obtained a rate of twenty-three cm. per hour. As compared with the vast amount of water evaporated by the leaves and green portions of living plants, the quantity consumed by the chemico-vital processes taking place in the cells during growth is trifling.

Among all the functions displayed by vegetable life, transpiration should, in point both of absorbing interest and practical value, be placed in the foremost rank. It undoubtedly is the physiological marvel as to activity, and yet it is a mysterious phenomenon, occurring in the vast majority of instances wholly beyond our limited powers of vision. It belongs to the organic functions (being common to the animal and vegetable kingdoms), and it mainly corresponds to the insensible perspiration from the human skin, though it shows much more energy than the latter process.

It is to be noted, however, that certain plants actually have, when well matured, been known to distil moisture drop by drop from the ends of their leaves. According to the Dutch anatomist Ruysch (quoted by Pouchet, *loc. cit.*), this phenomenon was observed in an Arum which he kept in a greenhouse in the Botanical Garden of Amsterdam. To confirm this remarkably curious case we may allude to the experiments of M. Ch. Musset, who has discovered that a plant of the same family, the edible Arum, launches little drops of water in the form of a jet into the air, and that these exhale from the pores which we see on the tips of its magnificent heart-shaped leaves, undulating like the waves of the sea. He tells us that from each of these orifices from ten to a hundred drops of water were thrown every minute the distance of an inch or more. But the so-called weeping tree (Cœsalpinia pluviosa), according to the account given by travellers through the Canary Islands, in this regard richly deserves the distinction bestowed upon it of "vegetable marvel," since it had, by numerous learned observers, been noticed to distil water "like copious rain from its tufted foliage." Though the vegetable kingdom under natural conditions presents but a limited number of instances of this extraordinary phenomenon, yet these are quite ample to serve to complete the parallel between the process as exhibited by plants and by animals, for it cannot be looked upon otherwise than as the exact counterpart of the sensible perspiration in the latter. The vast difference as to the rate of transpiration between the two kingdoms will hereafter become conspicuously apparent.

According to Pouchet (*loc. cit.*), for the idea that plants, like animals, transpire we are indebted to Mueschenbroeck, a former professor at the University of Leyden. He likewise gives us the following brief though interesting narrative of the ingenious experiments which led to the discovery of this important function. For this purpose Mueschenbroeck covered with a plate of lead the whole circumference of the root of a white poppy, so as to prevent the vapor of the earth from interfering with his experiment. The plant was then covered with a bell-glass cemented to the lead. After that, each morning when the naturalist came to visit the imprisoned plant he observed that even during the dryest nights its leaves were covered with an innumerable number of these drops of water, to which the name of dew is given, and that the sides of the glass themselves were quite obscured by it.

The first set of experiments worthy of mention performed with a view to attempt to estimate the rate of transpiration in plants are those of Guettard (quoted by Pouchet), who conceived the idea of enclosing a branch not separated from the plant in a globe of glass terminating outwardly in a neck which was inserted in a flask. Once all was hermetically sealed, it was found to be an easy task to collect without the slightest loss the exhaled moisture, which after condensing itself on the sides of the glass fell drop by drop into the bottle situated beneath the branch. It was found that a branch of a Cornel tree weighing only five drachms and a half, exhaled each day an ounce and three drachms of water; or the equivalent of twice its weight in twenty-four hours. Whilst this experiment gave really brilliant results, a truer idea of this functional energy would have been yet more astounding to this investigator, for it should be here noted that in his experiment there was no opportunity for the action of wind-currents, which, as will appear obvious hereafter, have an important influence in accelerating this process of nature. The result of the interesting observations of Garreau (*Annales des Sciences Nat.*, 3d ser., bot. xiii. 355) on the transpiration from single leaves doubtless should, considering the means employed, be accepted as thoroughly trustworthy. It will, however, be seen that while the results are of value as showing the connection between this process and the number of stomata, his experiments were, it seems to me, not made with the definitive purpose of reckoning the amount of exhalation from a given area of leaf-surface. He collected the exhaled moisture by means of chloride of calcium, placing the leaf between two bell-jars, one applied to its upper and the other to its under surface. His conclusions were: first, the quantity of water exhaled by the upper and under surfaces of the leaf is usually as 1 to 2, 1 to 3, or even 1 to 5 or more. The quantity has no relation to the position of the surfaces, for the leaves when reversed gave the same results as when in their natural position; secondly, there is a correspondence between the quantity of water exhaled and the number of stomata; thirdly, the transpiration of fluid takes place in greater quantity on the parts of the epidermis where there is the least waxy or fatty matter, as along the line of the ribs.

An ancient observer, Hales ("Statical Essays; Vegetable Statics," p. 21, quoted by Bessey), found that the amount of water exhaled from a vine in twelve hours of daylight equalled a film only .13 mm. (.005 in.) thick, and having an extent as great as that of the evaporating surface; the amount from a cabbage in the same time equalled a film .31 mm. (.012 in.) thick; from an apple-tree, .25 mm. (.01 in.) thick; from a sunflower in a day and night, equals a film .15 mm. (.006 in.) thick. From further calculations Hales concludes that the quantity of moisture exhaled from the sunflower with a leaf-surface 5616 square inches was from twenty to thirty ounces in twelve hours, being about seventeen times as rapid as man exhales. This plant during a clear night lost three ounces, but on a dewy night nothing.

In his work on botany Balfour (p. 457) refers to the researches of Woodward, giving some of the results of this observer. Woodward took plants and, having immersed their roots in water, placed them in the light for more than a month. He noticed the quantity absorbed and that transpired as well (making allowances for extraneous evaporation), and showed that the greater quantity of the water absorbed was again given off by the leaves. Inasmuch as these plants were, by allowing their roots to rest in pure water, placed under decidedly artificial conditions, it is questionable whether results thus obtained are much to be relied upon, for it is a known fact that certain plants (Calla Ethiopica for example) which ordinarily do not do so can, when moisture is too abundantly supplied to their roots, be made to distil the water from their leaves. In his agreeable experiments, Sachs, with a view to obtain fresh light upon the subject, employed the leaves of the white poplar, and found the rate of transpiration to be about one-third that from water, while on the other side Müller, with much less perseverance, found the rate to be only one-seventeenth as rapid as from water. Our readers doubtless will have noticed the great discrepancy in the results obtained by the various authorities cited, and since the question is really one of vital moment, such a state of things is regrettable in the extreme. Moreover, when the great practical importance of the subject is taken into account, it is not a little surprising to find that up to within a recent period the literature relating thereto should embrace such a paucity of reliable observations, since those recited consist for the most part of bare statements of results, and, curiously enough, in every instance in which experiments upon entire growing plants have been given in detail, the objectionable circumstance of exposing the plants to unnatural or interfering conditions has obtained.

It was doubtless owing in great measure to a full appreciation of the imperfection of previous methods that led our famous American botanist, Professor J. T. Rothrock, while lecturing some nine or ten years since to his class at the University of Pennsylvania upon the function in question, to remark the great importance of keeping the plants in a healthy normal state while being experimented with. To accomplish this it was suggested by him that something impervious to moisture should be adjusted to the receptacle in which the plant had previously been growing, so as to prevent any evaporation from the vessel or soil in which the plant was situated. The plant was now to be weighed at stated intervals, and the loss of weight in any given time would represent the weight of the liquid transpired. The importance of making a careful series of experiments in reference to transpiration was also strongly urged by the professor. The writer, at that time a member of the class which Professor Rothrock so ably and satisfactorily instructed, being strongly impressed by these opportune suggestions, determined to make an experimental study of the theme.

Experiments were forthwith instituted with the view, not only to ascertain as nearly as possible the amount of water exhaled by plants in a healthy natural state, but also to determine the connection between certain meteorological conditions and variations, the nature of the cortical tissue of the leaves and transpiration. The results of these experiments formed the basis of a graduation essay under the caption "Transpiration in Plants."* To accomplish the ends in view the following means were employed. A piece of good rubber cloth of sufficient size was taken, and its narrower border tucked up neatly around the base of the stem of the plant and secured by means of an elastic cord. The rubber cloth was then allowed to drop down over the vessel in which the plant was situated, the portion of the cloth underneath the pot gathered up and brought to one side of its base, and after giving it a few twists in one direction so as insure its close application to all parts of the pot, the twisted portion was well wrapped and tied off by means of a cord so as to keep it in this condition. This done, the line of separation at the point where the edges of the cloth met was remedied by allowing overlapping of two inches or more and sealing by means of gum mucilage. It was now thought that evaporation from the vessel was next to impossible, but the question next arose, "How is the plant to be supplied with the necessary moisture?" This difficulty was overcome by taking a hollow cylinder of tin three-fourths of an inch in diameter, about three inches in length, and having made a hole of sufficient size in the cloth covering the pot, a few inches from the stem of the plant, introducing one end of this tube into the opening, the rubber cloth was tucked up and tied on it the same as in

---

* This essay was presented to the faculty of the Auxiliary Department of Medicine of the University of Pennsylvania, and was awarded the George B. Wood Prize in 1877.

It was afterwards read before the Alumni Society of the Auxiliary Department, and under the auspices of that society was published in the *American Naturalist* for March, 1878.

the case of the stem of the plant, the external opening of the tube being guarded by means of a cork. To assert that this arrangement would allow of no escape of moisture whatever would be useless as well as illogical, yet there is perfect safety in affirming that, as compared with the amount transpired by the plant itself, the quantity lost sinks into insignificance. But we need not thus neglect this small loss, since it can be successfully offset against a trivial gain in another direction, namely, the slight increase in weight of the plant by the gases which it fixes during the time of a single experiment. Reflecting that plants return to the atmosphere the greater portion by volume of the gases absorbed by them, this must be considered very small indeed, though it is doubtless in excess of the loss of moisture by insecurity of our method, which loss certainly could not have exceeded a few grains per day. It is quite obvious that the mode adopted is not calculated to favor an overestimate of the rate of transpiration. Our plants were watered in the morning before weighing them for the day's experiment, and just sufficient water was supplied to keep them in a healthful state, the conditions of the leaves being in all cases taken as a guide. After watering the plants each morning they were carefully weighed, and then placed in the desired position, and left undisturbed till evening or any number of hours desired, and then were again weighed. The loss of weight, as before stated, was considered equivalent to the amount evaporated during the time of the experiments. Usually one observation was made for a day and a night, but the plants were also weighed in the evening, so as to establish the relation between day and night evaporation during the same twenty-four hours.

As before intimated, the relationship between the dew-point, temperature, etc., and the rapidity of transpiration was noted in most of the observations made. This was arrived at by means of the ordinary wet-bulb thermometer, taking the average temperature and dew-point according to the well-known rule, which it would be needless to detail here. With this brief yet, it is hoped, sufficiently comprehensive description of the method pursued, we shall turn to notice the results obtained by these experiments.

The first plant employed was a common calla (*Calla Æthiopica*), an herbaceous plant three feet one and a half inches high. Its whole weight on taking it up, with roots cleaned, was two pounds two ounces; weight of the evaporating portion, or all above ground, one pound three ounces, and two hundred and forty grains in a green state. It might be well to state here that in order to ascertain their weight the plants were taken up after the experiments were made upon them.

With the calla placed in the open air, the average loss of weight or its equivalent, the amount of water evaporated in twelve hours during the day, was about two thousand eight hundred and fifty grains, while in the in-door experiments in the same interval the rate was a little more than half as rapid. The important part played by the sun's rays and atmospheric currents is strongly indicated by the results from this plant. Thus, while in-doors it received the solar rays only about half the time during a clear day, and although the room in which it was kept was well ventilated, the currents were in no way comparable to the circulation of air outside. It was found, very curiously, that this plant exhaled nothing during a cloudy night, either within or out of doors, and during clear nights in open air, on the average only about four hundred and sixty grains.

The plant next chosen was our common geranium (*Pelargonium cucullata*). Also herbaceous; eighteen inches high; weight in a green state, with roots washed, nine ounces one hundred and twenty grains; of green or exhaling part, seven ounces. Not less striking than those with the calla were the results with this plant. They indicate that the amount exhaled at night is about the same in the open air as in the house, while the evaporation in daytime is more than double in the former what it is in the latter position,—a fact, it will be seen, which is slightly at variance with the results from the calla.

The average rate of transpiration for the geranium exceeded even that of the calla, being three thousand five hundred grains in twelve hours. It should be noted that this plant exhaled more than the weight of the portion with exhaling surface in the course of twenty-four hours. This and the previous plant, it should be remarked, were in the flowering stage.

A flowering fuchsia (*F. macrostemma*) was next employed, a shrubby plant whose leaf-surface we estimated at four hundred and fifty square inches; height of plant, twenty-seven inches; weight of the portion having evaporating surface, two ounces; of whole plant, with roots washed and in a green state, four ounces. Coincident with the remainder of the experiments, we made observations on the average temperature and dew-point. These latter observations, it should be observed, were taken in the same medium in which the plant was situated. The latter in the in-door experiments were, in all instances, placed about four feet from the window. This plant gave exceedingly interesting results. In these experiments the average temperature was higher and the dew-point correspondingly lower during the time of the observations made on this plant in the house than while exposed to the open air; this, no doubt, accounts for the fact that more moisture was lost at night while the plant was kept in-doors than when exposed, the average at night having been five hundred and forty grains while in-doors, and only four hundred and twenty grains outside. The temperature and the relative humidity of the atmosphere would therefore seem to influence transpiration even at night. As in the observations with previous plants, these results also showed that the process is at least twice as active during the day, when the plant was exposed, as when kept in the house; and yet we must not lose sight of the fact before mentioned, namely, that the average temperature and the average complement of the dew-point were higher during the experiments made in-doors than when the plant was out of doors. To the proposition that sunlight and currents of air are, one or both of them, powerful modifiers of this process, intelligent readers will give hearty assent. This plant, it is interesting to note, exhaled one hundred grains more than its own weight (four ounces) in twelve hours. To further confirm the effect of wind-currents upon transpiration, we may call attention to the fact that on the last day the fuchsia was experimented with rather strong winds prevailed, and while the temperature was no higher and the difference between the dry bulb and the dew-point was not as great as on the previous day, it was found to exhale most,— exceeding by ninety-two grains all the rest of the results. The hydrangea, which plant was next used, still better exemplified the influence of these currents, since it was found to exhale at least one ounce more during Experiment I. (a windy day, see table) than on any succeeding day. Apart from the influence of winds and given a clear day, a glance at the tables of results from the two last plants shows us a direct correspondence between the complement of the dew-point and the rate of transpiration in these cases. This latter fact will appear more evident hereafter. Upon the hydrangea a few observations were made with the view of determining the rate of evaporation of different periods during the day. It was found that while in the open air this plant transpired between the hours of 11 A.M. and 3 P.M. as much as in the remaining eight hours of the day's experiment.

Our fifth plant was a *Camellia japonica*, a shrubby plant twenty-eight inches high, with a leaf-surface of four hundred and seventy-nine inches. The results which this plant gave us exhibit in a satisfactory manner the connection between the character of the leaf-structure and the rapidity of evaporation. The fact that this plant had leaves of dense structure and with thick cortical coverings must account for the very much smaller quantity transpired, and yet some allowance ought to be made in this case for the less favorable meteorological conditions, as shown by the table (see *post*), during the time that the plant was used.

Again, it is quite probable that in plants with evergreen leaves having thick epidermal tissue transpiration is only possible through the stomata, whereas in the case of leaves which are thin, soft, and rapidly growing, with little cortical tissue, evaporation is more general from their surfaces. However this may be, the fact remains that the nature of the cuticular tissue is hereby shown to be closely related to the amount of liquid transpired.

The camellia exposed during a cloudy and dewy night gained, as is seen by the table, in weight to the extent of three hundred and ten grains; the same thing occurred on a rainy night in the house, when the plant was situated about four feet from an open window, the gain in the latter case being two hundred and thirty grains. This plant showed no loss by evaporation at night in the open air.

A lantana (*L. carnosa*), a shrubby plant, eighteen inches high, leaf-surface three hundred and thirty square inches, weighing only one and one-half ounces, was also employed. As compared to the extent of leaf-surface, this plant evaporated more than any other plant tried, reaching, on a clear windy day, nearly two ounces per square foot of leaf-surface in twelve hours. It was further observed to exhale nearly three times its own weight in twelve hours. The leaves of this little wonder were very thin and soft, a fact which may account for the remarkably rapid transpiration from their surfaces. With the lantana, as was done with the hydrangea, a few experiments were made to ascertain whether the process was more rapid about mid-day than at other periods or not. It was found to be most rapid about noon or a little after; and it was found here, also, that half the quantity evaporated by day was given off between the hours of 11 A.M. and 3 P.M. These observations were made on clear days.

The next or last growing plant used was a dracæna, an herbaceous plant with large leaves (being cultivated for its foliage). Its leaf-surface was estimated at eight hundred and seventeen square inches; its height twenty-seven inches.

In comparison to the extent of leaf-surface, this plant did not exhale as fast as most of the other plants used. The fact of the dracæna having smooth and more or less dense leaves doubtless accounts for the relatively less rapid evaporation. In the case of the two last plants tried it was particularly noticed, as in the two before them, that, other things being equal, dryness of the atmosphere was favorable to the process of transpiration. The favorable influence of winds over this process in plants was once more seen in the experiments with both the lantana and dracæna. The scales used in all our experiments were accurately adjusted.

The following tabular record of our results, which amply speak for themselves, are here inserted, with the hope that their scrutiny may prove of considerable interest to the student of science. We have deemed it prudent to premise each table by simply giving the name and area in square inches of evaporating surface of each plant.

HOUSE-PLANTS AS SANITARY AGENTS. 93

First Plant, Calla Æthiopica: Evaporating Surface not computed.

Experiment.	Duration of Experiment.	Loss of Weight or Amount Evaporated.	Place.	Weather.
I.	12 hours, day.	1420 gr.	In-doors.	Clear.
II.	" "	195 "	"	Cloudy, rain.
III.	" "	1440 "	"	Clear and warm.
IV.	" "	2040 "	In open air.	Partly cloudy.
V.	" "	2380 "	"	Clear.
VI.	" "	3320 "	"	Clear, windy.

Second Plant, Geranium (Pelargonium cucullata); Evaporating Surface not reckoned.

Experiment.	Duration of Experiment.	Loss by Evaporation.	Loss by Day, 12 Hours.	Place.	Weather.
I.	Day and night.	1560 gr.	1080 gr.	In-doors.	Clear.
II.	" "	1930 "	1440 "	"	"
III.		....	1286 "	"	"
IV.	Day and night.	3380 gr.	2880 "	In open air.	"
V.	" "	3730 "	3220 "	"	Clear, very warm.
VI.	" "	3390 "	2900 "	"	"

Third Plant, Fuchsia macrostemma; Exhaling Surface, 450 Square Inches.

Experiment.	Duration of Experiment.	Loss of Weight by Evaporation.	Loss by Day, Twelve Hours.	Average Temperature.	Average Dew-Point.	Place.	Weather.
		Gr.	Gr.				
I.	Day and night.	1810	1200	77°	61.4°	In-doors.	Clear.
II.	" "	1800	1240	72°	51.2°	"	"
III.	" "	1450	980	68°	49.9°	"	Partly cloudy.
IV.	" "	2270	1910	63.5°	49.5°	In open air.	Cloudy, some rain.
V.	" "	2415	1930	65.9°	50.5°	"	Clear, partly cloudy.
VI.	" "	2310	2020	65°	49.9°	"	Clear, windy.

94 HOUSE-PLANTS AS SANITARY AGENTS.

Fourth Plant, Hydrangea arborescens; presenting an Exhaling Surface of 744 Square Inches.

Experiment.	Place of Experiment.	Duration of Experiment.	Loss of Weight by Evaporation.	Loss by Day, Twelve Hours.	Average Temperature.	Average Dew-Point.	Weather.
I.	In open air.	Day and night.	Gr. 3010	Gr. 2450	71°	54.6°	Clear, windy.
II.	"	"	2395	1910	71°	55.8°	Clear, calm.
III.	"	"	2425	1940	75.5°	59.2°	Clear.
IV.	"	"	2415	2045	75°	57.5°	"
V.	In-doors.	"	1460	975	79°	58.7°	"
VI.	"	"	1370	900	80°	59.8°	"

Fifth Plant, Camellia japonica; Leaf Surface, 179 Square Inches.

Experiment.	Duration of Experiment.	Loss of Weight by Evaporation.	Loss by Day, Twelve Hours.	Average Temperature.	Average Dew-Point.	Place.	Weather.
I.	Day and night.	Gr. 710	Gr. 710	78.5°	63.3°	In open air.	Clear.
II.	" "	650	650	79.5°	71.3°	"	Cloudy, part, some rain.
III.	" "	170	480	70°	71.3°	"	Cloudy, clear at night.
IV.	" "	......	240	74°	63°	In-doors.	Cloudy.
V.	" "	10	190	74°	65.7°	"	Cloudy and rainy in part.
VI.	" "	250	250	74.5°	65.8°	"	Clear.

Sixth Plant, Lantana (L. carnosa); exhaled from an Area of 330 Square Inches.

Experiment.	Duration of Experiment.	Loss of Weight by Evaporation.	Loss by Day, Twelve Hours.	Average Temperature.	Average Dew-Point.	Place.	Weather.
I.	Day and night.	Gr. 1360	Gr. 1200	66°	52.2°	In open air.	Clear, cloudy.
II.	" "	988	988	64°	54.4°	"	Cloudy during day.
III.	" "	1820	1820	76°	63.3°	"	Clear, windy, dewy night.
IV.	" "	2120	1920	79.5°	65.6°	"	Clear, windy day.
V.	" "	......	1930	79°	66°	"	Clear, windy.

Seventh, or Last Plant, a Dracæna; Surface for Transpiration, 817 Square Inches.

Experiment.	Duration of Experiment.	Loss of Weight by Evaporation.	Loss by Day, Twelve Hours.	Average Temperature.	Average Dew-Point.	Place.	Weather.
I.	Day and night.	Gr. 2784	Gr. 2410	66°	52.2°	In open air.	Clear.
II.	" "	1870	1385	64°	54.4°	"	Cloudy, clear at night.
III.	" "	2601	2351	70°	63.3°	"	Clear during night.
IV.	" "	2670	2410	79.5°	66.6°	"	Clear, windy day, night.
V.	" "	2770	2520	79°	66°	"	Clear, much wind.

SUMMARY OF INVESTIGATIONS.

In clear weather, the evaporation by night as compared to that which takes place in the day appears to be about in the ratio of 1 to 5. In some cases no loss occurred on dewy or cloudy nights. The camellia, however, lost nothing during clear nights and gained in weight on dewy or rainy nights, even when kept indoors. Under ordinary circumstances, transpiration at night was about the same in-doors as in the open air.

The true rate of transpiration during the day showed a very different relation, giving a ratio of 2 to 1 in favor of the open air. Of the whole amount exhaled during twelve hours of the day experiments, half was given off between the hours of 11 A.M. and 3 P.M., as shown by repeated testing.

The following, compiled for the number of clear days, will serve to exhibit the average rate of out-door transpiration which took place by day during clear weather. It will also show the relation between leaf-surface and the weight of the plant and the amount transpired. The mean temperature and average dew-point have been recorded as well.

Experiment.	Name of Plant.	Duration of Experiment.	Average Evaporation.	Evaporating Surface.	Weight of Plant.	Average Temperature.	Average Dew-Point.
		Hours.	*Gr.*				
I.	Calla.	12	2850	All plants green.	2 lbs. 2 oz.	......	......
II.	Geranium.	12	3500	"	4120 gr.	......	......
III.	Fuchsia.	12	1975	450 sq. in.	1920 "	64.5°	49 6°
IV.	Hydrangea.	12	2858	744 "	2170 "	73°	56 7°
V.	Camellia.	12	710	479 "	......	75.5°	63.3°
VI.	Lantana.	12	1717½	330 "	720 gr.	75.1°	61.7°
VII.	Dracæna.	12	2422	817 "	......	75.5°	62°

After an inspection of this table, our readers could easily compute for themselves the average rate of transpiration, which would be found to be about one and one-quarter ounces per day (twelve hours) for every square foot of leaf-surface. The lantana shows nearly two ounces to the square foot of surface. The camellia, with its dense, smooth leaves, averages less than half an ounce to the square foot of surface per day.

Although this rate is somewhat at variance with the results arrived at by most of the authors previously cited (*supra*), the fact deserves to be again mentioned that experiments carefully conducted with the apparatus used in the present series, in which the plants were, without creating the slightest artificial condition, kept vigorously growing, could scarcely admit of error in the results. To confirm more fully our conclusions upon the significant point in question, it may be briefly told that in an interesting series of experiments subsequently performed with the purpose of drawing comparisons between the rate of transpiration from known areas of leaf, land, and water surfaces, and employing the same methods, the results were entirely concordant. In the papers containing an account of the latter experiments the following statement, among others of like character, may be found : for fourteen consecutive days of clear and partly cloudy weather the mean transpiration for the plant (a small geranium, exposing, as nearly as could be calculated, one square foot of surface) was a little more than one and a quarter ounces per day. So far as our experiments relate to the rate of transpiration, the results throughout were quite unexpected, and our readers will doubtless concede their great value and interest in revealing to us the amazing energy residing in this occult process of nature.

To refer again to our researches, it may be seen by comparing the results from the camellia with those from other plants having soft thin leaves, that the peculiarities of leaf-structure among the agencies modifying the rate of transpiration stand paramount. The experiments of Garreau, before referred to, it is to be particularly observed in an especial degree lend support to this important deduction. His demoustration of the point that there is a correspondence between the amount of water exhaled by a plant and the number of stomata in its leaves, receives rather striking confirmation in the decision we rendered relative to the rate of exhalation from the camellia, inasmuch as it has been experimentally shown by other observers that plants whose leaves are dents and covered by a thick cuticle have fewer stomata than thin-leaved plants. To suppose, however, that in the case of soft, thin leaves this correspondence between the quantity transpired and the number of stomata is a strict one, must, in view of the strong probability already pointed out,— namely, that the latter leaves exhale from their general surfaces,—be far from correct. Thus far we have been speaking principally of the transpiration from foliar or green organs, but it should be added when, as usually obtains in older branches and the trunks of trees, the cortical tissue is a thick coating of bark, we find the exhalation from these organs is infinitesimal. Apart from anatomical formation, the sun's rays doubtless stand first among the exciting or modifying influences, for, going back to the results from the fuchsia, for instance, we find the average transpiration and dew-point higher during the in-door experiments than when the plant was exposed, and yet the relations of transpiration in the two situations were, other things being equal, about as ordinarily the case. In the case of the hydrangea the same thing obtained to a still more marked degree.

In the sequential series of experiments conducted, to which brief allusion has been made, there is also a striking confirmation of this view. One of our conclusions there reached having a direct bearing, it will be adduced. It was found that while the evaporation from this soil was greatly influenced by temperature and the degree of humidity, for the mean temperature and dew-point were both recorded in all these experiments, transpiration was in a marked degree excited by the direct rays of the sun. Not less valuable is the observation pointed out by the venerable editor of the science column of the *New York Independent*, Mr. Thomas Mechan, who tells us that our demonstration of the work intrusted to the solar rays relative to this function is in exact accordance with Deherain's discovery, of which we previously had been entirely ignorant,—that, while heat causes evaporation from dead organic matters, light is the great agent in transpiration in living vegetation.

Since the results from all of our direct experiments have been found to evidence the truth of the hypothesis here brought forward, we naturally have formed a strong opinion in its favor, and this while fully alive to the fact that not a few noted vegetable physiologists are unwilling to sanction the idea of attributing so decisive an effect to the action of the sun's rays, notwithstanding. In this connection it is well to note that in his "Text-Book of Botany," p. 602, the illustrious Sachs holds it to be doubtful whether light, that is, radiation, as such, independently of the elevation of temperature caused by it, influences transpiration.

Another controlling influence of considerable potency is exercised by the wind-currents. It was observed, however, that in cloudy days strong currents of air did not raise the daily quantity of vapor exhaled to the same extent as on clear days, and there is an obvious explanation of the fact that currents are more efficacious to hasten the process on the latter than on the former days. In clear weather the sunlight has the effect to open wide the stomata or pores in the leaves, thus naturally facilitating the escape of the aqueous vapor, which the atmospheric currents would in turn remove as it is formed, and thus really act as a *vis à fronte* to the vaporizing fluid within. Of the influence of currents, then, it may be said that in clear weather they are very effective in favoring the process, in cloudy weather their influence is less noticeable. On clear days strong currents increased the amount over that of calmer days by about one-fifth or even one-fourth. That elevation of temperature and the degree of saturation of the air are agencies which have an effect upon this phenomenon is indisputable, but there is little doubt that their rank, in point of potency, is subordinate to sunlight. It should be remarked, however, as a fact worthy of record, that in every instance tried in our researches, other things being considered, the complement of the dew-point or dryness had the effect to modify considerably the rate of transpiration, and, strange as it may appear, this seemed to be, in great measure at least, independent of the temperature.

A few calculations deduced from our experiments may serve to impress the importance of the ratio of transpiration. According to the above rate, the Washington elm at Cambridge, a tree it is stated of no very large size, with its two hundred thousand square feet of leaf-surface in twelve hours of clear weather transpires not less than seven and three-fourths tons of watery vapor. Carrying the calculation a single step further, a grove consisting of five hundred trees, each with a leaf-surface equal to that of the elm mentioned, would in twelve hours return to the atmosphere three thousand nine hundred tons of aqueous vapor. Even supposing this to be overestimated, from the facts of the case, it may be concluded *a priori* that the evaporation from growing plants is a powerful agent in maintaining a proper degree of moisture in the surrounding medium. Verily, to plants may be assigned honorable rank as natural and perfect atomizers, making their influence everywhere felt beyond question. At the conclusion of the paper from which the foregoing facts relative to transpiration have in the main been taken, we have ventured to suggest the practical value of keeping living plants in occupied rooms, in which the air is generally dryer than outside.

The latter observation, it will be seen, is, to speak in all modesty, pregnant with important suggestions of a peculiarly practical character.

It is but natural to suppose such thoughts should have the effect to open up to the mental eye a new field for further experimental research, and one of leading interest to the hygienist. Indeed, having explored the function of transpiration in its relations both to special causation and functional activity, it seemed to be urgently needful to follow up this subject by making the attempt to reduce to more practical knowledge what had already been gained by actual experiments. Knowledge of any sort whatever, it should be recollected, is of little real value except it is found to bear the test of applied scientific methods. Hence, to demonstrate whether or not plants on account of their transpiratory function could be employed for hygienic purposes in the home, experiments were instituted.

These researches, that we now purpose to present in detail, brought out some striking as well as encouraging facts, which clearly established a claim for the practical utility of the effects of transpiration in plants, and it is a little surprising that up to the date of the appearance of the article embracing a full account (see "Beneficial Influence of Plants," *Am. Nat.*, Dec. 1878) of these experiments sanitarians failed to draw attention to its significance as a means of overcoming the ill effects of the dry atmosphere of our dwellings. Almost at the very outset of this article we have presumed to make the proposition—a deduction from actual experiment—that the hygienic conditions of the air are both directly and indirectly affected by plant transpiration. The statement ventured, it is seen, contains two distinct elements, the one implying the direct effect of transpiration on the quantity of moisture in the atmosphere, the other the indirect. The direct effect of this process may be formulated thus: in all atmospheres in which the proportion of aqueous vapor is less than the healthiest standard, about seven-eighths of what the air can contain at a given temperature, the beneficial influence of transpiration must be measured by the amount exhaled from the plants. In this connection the fact so forcibly brought out by the rather brilliant results of our experiments with reference to transpiration (*loc. cit.*) should not be lost sight of, namely, that the process during the day is only about half as active in-doors as in the open air, but the rate at night is about similar in the two situations, so that the quantity a plant would during the whole twenty-four hours exhale on the interior exceeds half what it would give off on the exterior.

To the end of showing conclusively the exact ability of plants to augment the degree of moisture in closed rooms, we will now for the sake of clearness draw from this paper a copious extract.

From observations which, thanks to the courtesy of the superintendent, Dr. S. R. Knight, we were privileged to make over a period of several weeks on the air of our private reading- and sleeping-room at the Episcopal Hospital (Philadelphia), which is kept warm by air heated by steam, and simultaneously on the air outside, we found the air in the former position to be appreciably dryer than in the latter, the average complement of the dew-point being on the whole about five degrees greater. The room adjoining mine, occupied by my colleague, was very kindly left for a time at my disposal. In it were kept a few thrifty-growing plants in pots, with a leaf-surface of not more than twelve square feet. The dimensions of the room were similar, each being twenty feet long, eleven feet wide, and sixteen feet high, each having one window fronting east, in which the plants were kept. The average temperature and dew-point in both these rooms were noted simultaneously, and the results showed uniformly for a period of eighteen days that the complement of the dew-point averaged one and a half degrees less in the room containing the plants. These observations were made during the early part of April, 1878, when very little heat was required, still the windows were kept closed during the day. Calculating from these results the effect of twenty-four square feet of leaf-surface on the air of a room half the size of the above would be to increase sufficiently the humidity to raise the dew-point six degrees Fahrenheit,—higher than it would be if there were no plants in the room.

As it seemed possible that the variation in the amount of moisture in the two rooms tested might be due to considerations other than the presence of plants, it was deemed necessary to vary the conditions and make further observations. Accordingly, after placing some plants—about the same number as were used in the experiments above narrated—in the window of my own room, I took the average temperature and dew-point and compared them with those of an adjoining room containing no plants. No artificial heat was required during the time of these experiments. It was found that when the window was kept open so as to cause very free ventilation no appreciable difference in the results from the two rooms was observed, but if the windows, on the other hand, were closed for a few (say three) hours, it would make a difference of from one and a half to two degrees Fahr. in the complement of the dew-point; the room having plants showing the lesser complement. This difference was almost maintained when the windows were opened just enough to allow a gradual interchange of the contained air; but, as before intimated, a draught, though it might hasten transpiration, would, by carrying off the vapor, prevent any increase of moisture in the air of the room. On days when the air was laden with moisture no difference in the dew-point was noticed, there being at such times little or no exhalation of watery vapor. The observations taken at 1 o'clock P.M. gave the greatest variation, the morning observations usually the least. We do not wish to say, dogmatically, that there is no possible chance of error in these experiments, but since they were throughout corroborative, it seems fair to conclude that they are correct. Since it is always allowable to make logical deductions from known facts, we may from the statements above made concerning the rate of transpiration, coupled with the carefully conducted observations here detailed, justly conclude that during the summer months, when the windows are thrown widely open and the doors kept ajar, the influence of transpiration is quite inconsiderable; on the other hand, when the interchange of air is not too rapid, a sufficient number of growing plants, well watered, have the effect (if the air be not already saturated) of increasing the moisture to any desirable extent.

Assuming, furthermore, that transpiration is to a much greater extent controlled by the action of the sun's rays than by the temperature range or the relative humidity of the atmosphere, then this process of nature must in clear weather, including the cold season, be more uniformly operated than evaporation from water or other sources under similar conditions. Of the latter fact there can be little room for doubt, since it is once more substantially corroborated by the results of observations which will be hereafter detailed. To the sanitarian the point here made presents a practical phase of paramount interest. In the first place the temperature is to some extent affected by the proportion of moisture the air contains, or, in other words, moistening the air has the effect slightly to lower the temperature. Changes in the degree of saturation, therefore, necessarily entail variations in the temperature; and applying these truths to the air of our dwellings, the obvious advantage of plant-moisture, which is more equally supplied, would be to secure on its part a more uniform temperature of the respirable medium in which we spend the greater portion of our lives. Of course, closely associated with this point is that which relates to the quantity of moisture essential to good health. At the ordinary temperature of living-rooms, say from 65° to 70° Fahr., the degree of humidity most conducive to health as well as most agreeable to the average individual is, as before incidentally stated, about seventy-five per cent. of saturation. This proportion, be it remembered, never obtains in our dwellings. It should here be remarked that, in our experiments, the relative humidity for the same temperature was found to be quite variable. To consider for a moment these facts in relation to the process of evaporation from the human body cannot fail to prove interesting to our readers. In the first place, if in an atmosphere of the proper temperature and proper standard of humidity the rate of evaporation from our bodies is the most healthy, then decidedly less moisture would increase the rate of exhalation to a point beyond the health limit, lowering at the same time the body temperature. Again, as all artificially heated atmospheres contain not only far too little moisture, but also exhibit marked variations, the evident effect upon our bodies is to cause excessive and variable evaporation. To increase the difficulty, there is the influence of temperature upon the phenomena of transpiration from the human body. That as its temperature rises the capacity of the air for moisture becomes to a proportionate degree increased, is a well-known hygienic axiom; hence it is obvious that a high temperature greatly enhances the evaporative action of the skin. Placing the body in a hot-air bath at a temperature of 160° to 140° Fahr. has, as physicians well know, the effect to cause the body to break out in copious perspiration. But in health such an effect is undesirable. On the other hand it is found that, even at the temperature of living-rooms, and more particularly when artificial heat is employed, illimitable mischief is the result.

Under such circumstances the temperature of the body must be at times suddenly reduced to the extent of causing sensations of chilliness to be experienced. To the truth of this proposition doubtless many of our readers would not be unwilling to give hearty approbation. Indeed, we may, in a conservative spirit, speaking from the stand-point of the practising physician, affirm that colds ordinarily so called,—catarrhal forms of inflammation of the mucous membranes of the head and air-passages,—and even graver forms of illness frequently have been found to be attributable to the same cause. Upon the invalid words are inadequate to express the effect of an atmosphere such as above depicted.

Respecting both the temperature and the degree of saturation, then, the quality of equanimity is more than ordinarily important, the effect being to assure a more nearly uniform rate of evaporation from the human frame. This circumstance would avert the necessity for the body to adapt itself to the more or less frequent and abrupt vicissitudes of temperature and humidity generally experienced in dwellings. According to the teachings of the very highest authorities in modern sanitary science, small daily fluctuations in the temperature, and, we may properly add, the relative humidity, are, so far as relates to the public health, of more vital moment than the general average of these meteorological elements over long periods of time.

But the most significant bearing of the results from our experiments is their application to the atmosphere of apartments heated by means of hot-air furnaces, for the excellent reason that such an atmosphere is known to be dryer than one heated by a stove or open fireplace or steam. Not having the opportunity myself at the Episcopal Hospital of comparing the dryness of the air thus warmed with that of the outer air, my wants were made known to a friend living in a house heated by a furnace. Through the kindness of this friend reliable observations for a period of eight consecutive days were made. The results showed the mean average complement of the dew-point to be seven degrees higher for the heated air than the air outside. Now, according to our previous line of reasoning, a certain number of house-plants would bring up the humidity of a chamber heated by dry air to that of the external air. Calculating from the above experimental data, half a dozen plants, 'each with a leaf-surface of six square feet, would be in a room twelve feet long and ten feet wide, with a ceiling twelve feet high, ample to produce this effect. But admitting that to meet the demand for moisture in such rooms twice or even thrice this number of plants would be in some instances required, have we not here a most charming means, now that all traditional alarm as to their supposed injurious influence has been removed, of furnishing moisture in the most acceptable form? With regard to the signal value of house-plants in such instances, a commentary is scarcely needful. It seems to me proper, however, to point out to the non-professional reader what are the specific effects upon the healthy individual produced by dry-air heat. It will be necessary to answer this inquiry only so far as relates to the effect of furnace heat at the ordinary temperature of occupied rooms. It will be at once evident that such an atmosphere would have the effect to hasten to an inordinate degree the exhalations from the skin. The mucous membranes of the head and air-passages become notably dried, frequently inducing irritation of those organs. By and by the mucous lining of the alimentary canal becomes unduly parched; thirst and loss of appetite being in this manner induced. Undoubtedly that prevailing and much to be dreaded habit of body, constipation, is not infrequently, owing to a lack of moisture in the intestines, in like manner produced. The urine is lessened in amount and is highly colored. Nor does the nervous system escape the deleterious effects of dry furnace heat. To show that such reasoning is not a mere fantasy on our part, we can adduce high authority; thus, that illustrious American author Professor A. Stillé ("Therapeutics," vol. i. pp. 637–38) gives us the following description of the injurious consequences of dry furnace heat. He writes, "If an apartment is heated to sixty-five or sixty-eight degrees Fahr., a person in good health and in ordinary clothing feels comfortable and experiences no immediate inconvenience. But the air contains a much smaller proportion of vapor than if the air were warmed to the same degree by a stove or open fireplace. In this manner a great demand is made upon the system to supply the air with moisture, the skin and pulmonary mucous membranes are dried, and a condition is induced which is expressed in irritability of the nervous system, paleness, and susceptibility of the skin to cold, liability to pulmonary diseases, and, in a word, deterioration of all the functions." Indeed, the circumstance of so large a portion of the population of large cities and towns using the hot-air furnace as a means of warming their dwellings would seem to justify the belief that there is a more or less immediate connection between the bodily ills of the inhabitants and this method of heating. That there are, on the other hand, good uses of dry forms of heat for the relief of a few diseases cannot be disputed, but it requires to be judiciously applied; in short, dry heat should be employed for sanitary purposes only under the direction of a skilled physician. If, as we have demonstrated, a proper number of house-plants grown in an apartment heated by dry air would have the effect of raising the percentage of vapor to the standard compatible with the best health, then the mission of cultivated plants as health-promoting agents cannot on this ground alone fail to receive the sanction of every practically-minded person, since under these circumstances they may become the means of obviating many distressing symptoms, or even actual disease. It is proper to mention here what has perhaps already suggested itself to the mind of the reader, that a larger amount of plant growth is required wherever artificial heating is accomplished by means of a furnace than by other means. To see them taking such high rank as sanitary agencies must be to all lovers of plants and flowers a source of intense gratification. At its very birth, then, this novel idea of the sanitary value of transpiration for the comfort and welfare of mankind promises much. Meanwhile, the writer hopes that the arguments up to this point put forward may also have the happy effect to heighten popular appreciation of these truly adorable objects of nature.

CHAPTER V.

Ozone—General statements relating thereto—Various modes of generating ozone—Do plants possess the power to generate it?—Experimental investigation of the question—Description of the tests for ozone—The first observations conducted in Horticultural Hall, Fairmount Park, Philadelphia—Description of same—Later experiments with glass case—In-door and out-door experiments, with odorous and non-odorous flowers—Conclusions drawn from the results obtained—A reinvestigation of the subject—Similar methods employed—The results with the flowers identical—Experiments with odorous foliage—Interesting results from the use of pine foliage—The nature of this ozone-generating process discussed—Facts and experiments by others corroborating our own conclusions—Sanitary value of ozone—The value of flowering plants as purifiers of the air of dwellings, which is usually abominable—Sources of house air impurities—House-plants as health-giving agents—Moral influences of plants and flowers—Review of sanitary relation of growing plants—Amount of plant life necessary for ordinary sanitary purposes.

As heretofore incidentally mentioned, there is carried on by plants another process which brings them into hygienic importance, namely, the generation of ozone. Up to a very recent period the subject has remained experimentally unexplored.

Nevertheless in my readings, while preparing earlier memoirs on some plant-functions, I would very rarely meet with statements to the effect that some sort of relationship exists between vegetation, and particularly forest growth, and the ozonic condition of the atmosphere. Thus, as elsewhere stated, a Dr. Schreiber maintains that the emanations from the pine foliage convert the oxygen of the air into ozone, but upon what basis of proof, if any, the statement rests we have not learned.

A French writer, A. Naquet, tells us "ozone exists in woods and fields, and wherever there is active vegetation." Assertions like the above of a general character without experimental proof, are obviously of no real scientific value. On the other hand, the solution of so important a question as whether plants generate, or convert the oxygen of the air into, ozone cannot fail to be hailed as a noteworthy advance in scientific knowledge.

Excepting such as have received the benefit of the higher medical education, including chemists and those who occupy themselves with the thankless task of working out problems for the public good, there has been little or no attention bestowed upon the atmospheric constituent known as ozone. Indeed, of the very existence of this substance not a small proportion of the thinking masses in general have been totally ignorant. Very recently, however, we have received fresh evidence of the unceasing spirit of scientific progress abroad in the fact that ozone, on the part of rival experimentalists, has been and is exciting a lively interest among leading hygienists, and if the quality of practical usefulness is to be regarded as a criterion of the practical value of an agent, then ozone, as will be seen hereafter, fully merits the attention that is now bestowed upon it. In general terms, than ozone there is no substance of higher importance to the sanitarian for study and consideration, since it has undoubted hygienic bearings, some of which are now pretty well understood. There is no question but that through its oxidizing properties it is the greatest natural purifier of the atmosphere. But concerning its special value as a sanitary agent more will hereafter be said. Meanwhile we shall present to our readers an account of two sets of experiments, which were conducted with a view of discovering whether or not growing plants really possess the power of furnishing to the atmosphere this valuable body. The first series of experiments were published in a succession of two articles under the title "The Exhalation of Ozone by Flowering Plants" (*Amer. Naturalist* for April and May, 1884). Without offering an apology for what may strike the reader as tedious details, these essays, with slight alterations in diction for prudential reasons, are here incorporated. It is true we have little certain knowledge of the real nature and many of the properties of ozone, and we cheerfully leave these more puzzling questions to the expert chemist. It can, however, be artificially formed in various ways, to wit: by passing an electric discharge through pure oxygen; by the electrolytic decomposition of water; by suspending a stick of phosphorus in a bottle filled with moist air, and in other ways. It is present in the atmosphere, but not universally. Fresh, pure atmosphere generally contains ozone, while it is absent from the close air of cities and occupied dwellings, for the reason that in the latter places it is consumed in oxidizing and destroying organic impurities. For a like reason it is frequently found in the air to the windward of a city, but rarely or never to the leeward.

For more than a year the writer, while engaged in the active practice of his profession, has devoted his intervals of leisure to an experimental investigation of the subject.

Preliminary to giving in detail the results of these experiments, it is thought proper to speak of the various tests for the detection of ozone, and to point out the relative merits of the same. As indicative of the difficulties of making such tests, numerous ozonoscopes have from time to time been devised, most of which have proved highly unsatisfactory.

An investigation into the relative merits of some half-dozen leading tests for ozone has been made by Dr. A. R. Leeds, of Stevens' Institute of Technology (see *Chemical News* for May, 1878). Without giving a detailed account of his observations, it will suffice our purpose to state a few of his conclusions. The Schönbein or oxidized starch test was found to be most sensitive. It may be here stated that this test was used in all our observations. Of the guaiacum test, which was also used in our experiments, Dr. Leeds remarks: "Guaiacum papers were only moderately sensitive, acquiring speedily, when dry, a faint blue color, and when moistened occupying a position midway between the ozonoscopes most sensitive and those least so to the influence of ozone."

In the *National Board of Health Bulletin* (for March, 1882) Dr. J. H. Long, under the auspices of the American Medical Association, records the results of ozone observations made in different places throughout the United States by a number of gentlemen who kindly co-operated with him. In these investigations three kinds of test-papers were employed, to wit: Schönbein paper, paper impregnated with tincture of guaiacum, and paper impregnated with solution of thallous hydrate.

The doctor gives the methods of preparing these different papers. The Schönbein is made according to the following formula: Potassium iodide 5 parts, starch 3 parts, and water 1000 parts. The starch and iodide are rubbed with a small amount of water until a milky homogeneous fluid is produced, and then the rest of the water is added and the whole boiled for some time with constant stirring. The freshly prepared paste is spread on strips of filter-paper, which are afterwards dried in a close room. The filter-paper used is the best Swedish (Murktell's). The guaiacum is made from a carefully prepared tincture containing eight per cent. of resin and ninety per cent. of alcohol; when exposed to artificially prepared ozone this paper turns greenish-blue and finally a bright blue, while the Schönbein turns quite blue.

The papers employed in the present researches were very kindly prepared for me by Professor Henry Leffmann after the above formulæ, and they gave excellent reactions both in the hands of the professor and in my own when exposed to ozone artificially prepared. The iodized starch, or Schönbein, being universally acknowledged to be the most sensitive as well as giving the most reliable results, the reactions obtained by this test were considered of paramount importance and value. There are, however, sometimes present in the atmosphere other bodies which have the power of destroying iodide of potassium, and hence give a blue reaction as well as ozone, namely, peroxide of hydrogen, the oxides of nitrogen and ammonia. The presence of the latter substance can be detected by suspending a piece of red litmus near the test-papers, the effect being to turn the litmus-paper blue. The presence of the nitrous oxides can also be readily demonstrated. How to avoid mistaking the reaction of peroxide of hydrogen for ozone may prove difficult, since the two substances appear to have many properties in common. Indeed, it has been a disputed question among chemists whether it is possible to distinguish between them by any known tests.

Professor A. R. Leeds (*Chem. News* for April 9, 1880) claims to be able to recognize each by its own properties. He continues: "The most striking property of ozone is its smell. This smell, so far as long-continued familiarity with it enables me to judge, whether the ozone is derived from the silent discharges of purer and dry oxygen, or accompanies the electrolysis of water (and the smell is identical), is possessed by ozone only." This odor is not peculiar to the peroxide of hydrogen. He adds: " Ozone is only slightly soluble in water, and is readily expelled in heating, while hydrogen peroxide is mixable, and solutions containing one per cent. of peroxide of hydrogen may be concentrated by evaporation on the water-bath until a higher degree of concentration is reached without great loss of peroxide." (See also Schöne, *Ann. der Chem.*, 196, p. 60, and Davis, *Chem. News*, vol. xxiv. p. 221.)

The question, can ozone and peroxide of hydrogen co-exist in the same atmosphere? has also been oppositely discussed by chemists. As the result of his investigations Professor McLeod (*Chem. News*, vol. xi. p. 307) concluded that these two bodies decompose one another. From this fact he further argues that it is extremely improbable that ozone and peroxide of hydrogen are both formed during the slow oxidation of phosphorus. On the other hand, Schöne, by an elaborate series of experiments (quoted by Leeds), shows that when strongly oxidized peroxide containing 5.2 volumes per cent. of ozone is agitated with an hydrogen peroxide solution containing 0.4 per cent. of the peroxide, or three or four times as much as is necessary to destroy all the ozone, it is only after the lapse of half an hour that as much as half of the ozone is destroyed. Professor Leeds in the article already referred to comes to the rescue of Schöne, and very conclusively shows that not only ozone, but peroxide of hydrogen is formed during the slow oxidization of phosphorus, and that these two substances can and frequently do coexist, the absolute quantity depending upon the temperature, the length of time they remain in contact with one another, etc., though it is true that when together a slow mutual decomposition takes place. According to all the best authorities, peroxide of hydrogen decomposes at a temperature of about 70° Fahr., while to destroy ozone requires a temperature of about 200° Fahr. The importance of this fact cannot be overrated, since it has a direct bearing upon the results of the present experiments.

In the case of the guaiacum test, there are so many interfering conditions as to render it nearly valueless. Thus, it will not only react in the presence of peroxide of hydrogen and the oxides of nitrogen, but even the oxygen of the atmosphere is also said to impart to it a tint hard to distinguish from the coloration due to ozone.

The color scales were not used in these researches, as they are very difficult to obtain, and furthermore our object was not so much to ascertain the degree of coloring of the test-papers as the single important fact whether or not growing plants possess the power to develop ozone.

In noting the results obtained, the terms "Marked," "Slight," and "Very slight" are used to express, in a general way, the extent of blue coloration. This plan was deemed preferable for the reason that the tints in most instances were not very striking.

My first observations were conducted in Horticultural Hall, Fairmount Park, Philadelphia. It was our belief that a careful testing of the air of this hall, filled as it is with a profusion of plants mostly of the foliage varieties, would give results sufficiently striking to be of value in clearing up the subject. In this, however, we were, as will be seen hereafter, measurably disappointed. This hall has several compartments. The so-called main hall is of about the following dimensions: two hundred and twenty feet in length, one hundred feet in width, and the dome-like roof being of glass in the centre, sixty-five feet high. The room is filled with a variety of species of palms, bananas, monsteras, colocasias, calladiums, ferns, bamboo canes, Australia and New Zealand pines, the *Ficus elastica*, and numbers of smaller foliage varieties.

Average temperature of the hall during the time of experiments, 70° Fahr.

On either side of the main hall are several smaller ones in which the air was likewise tested, known under the names fern-house, forcing-house, temperate-house, propagating-house, and economic-house. The dimensions of these rooms were, length one hundred feet, width thirty feet, ceiling curvilinear and of glass, twenty feet in height. The temperate-house contained half-hardy plants, as the orange, lemon, hibiscus, and a number of azaleas in bloom. The forcing-house contained bedding plants, geraniums, coleus, and achyranthes, but few blooming, mostly cuttings. The economic-house contained pitcher-plants, tea, coffee, chocolate, sugar, yuccas, cinchona, and aromatic plants. The propagating-house is located outside of the main building, and contained geraniums in bloom. The fern-house was well stocked with ferns. The average temperature of these apartments was as follows: economic-house, 80°; temperate-house, 55°; fern-house, 65°; forcing-house, 75° Fahr.

The first experiments were commenced October 14, 1882, and continued until the end of November. The atmosphere of the main hall was tested on twenty-five days, during which period the Schönbein gave negative results except on November 29 and 30, when this paper showed a "slight" blue tint. The papers were placed on the branches of the highest plants, moistened both when they were suspended and after being taken down, and the duration of the experiments varied from four to twenty-four hours. The guaiacum test-paper showed a "very slight" reaction for about one-half of these observations, but unfortunately this test could not be relied upon, while the tests with the Schönbein paper were too meagre on which to base conclusions. A few tests during this series were made simultaneously in the forcing- and fern-houses, with negative results.

These experiments, it should be stated, were conducted at a time when numerous visitors were daily attracted to the hall by the indescribable beauty of the plants, and hence it was thought not unreasonable to suppose that any ozone which might have been generated by the plants was consumed in oxidizing the organic matter given to the air by the visitors, since, as before pointed out, ozone is for similar reasons never detectable in the atmosphere of occupied dwellings. Though these experiments were barren of results, when we take into account the above circumstances they were not much to be wondered at.

The next series of observations were begun in the latter part of February, 1883, and were continued through the months of March and April. During the month of February there was an occasional visitor admitted; in March there were likewise very few, while in April the number was considerably greater, though not by any means numerous. These experiments yielded results somewhat more encouraging. The atmosphere on the exterior was simultaneously tested for the sake of comparison. The observations in the main hall were taken for fourteen days, Schönbein papers being used, and five of these gave "very slight" reaction, while the outer air during the same time gave six "very slight" reactions and one "slight." Twenty-four tests of the air in the temperate-house with the Schönbein gave only three "very slight" reactions. During these observations the outer air was tested twelve times, with but two "slight" reactions, and, for the remaining days in place of the outer air, the air of the propagating-house, which gave us two "very slight" reactions. The air of the propagating-house was next compared with the external air. For thirteen days in the former situation Schönbein paper gave "very slight" reactions in four instances, while the latter (outer air) in two instances gave "very slight" indications of ozone. It will be observed that here the result was better in the propagating-house than in the open air,—a fact which was, to say the least, quite suggestive. In all of the preceding experiments of this series there was a striking similarity in the two situations, the outer air giving somewhat the better results. The air of the fern-house, as well as that of the economic-house, was also given a few trials and compared with the outer air, but the results were negative throughout. During all of the out-door observations the guaiacum-paper in more than half of the experiments gave "slight" indications of ozone, and in four cases "marked." With this paper the results for corresponding days in-doors were almost identical, with the degree of coloring in a few instances in favor of the outside. The propagating-house yielded the best indoor results with the guaiacum-paper, as it did with the Schönbein, while the temperate-house gave results equally as good from the use of guaiacum-paper as in the propagating-house. This was not the case, it will be remembered, with the Schönbein. The duration of the individual experiments varied from six to sixteen hours, the average duration being about ten hours.

The question, Were the reactions obtained by the indoor tests due to ozone emitted from the plants or to the circulation of the outer air through the apartments?

here arises. There is constantly more or less interchange of air between the exterior and interior of the building, due to the numerous interstices between the panes of glass and the frequent opening and closing of the doors. It must also be noted that all of the apartments are heated (artificial heat being necessary during these experiments) by numerous hot-water pipes placed directly under and parallel with a grated floor, from which warm air arises and ascends through the building. The idea that the external conditions might have affected the results on the inside doubtless is still further strengthened by the fact that in part the results obtained were, as already stated, nearly identical in the two situations, with a preponderance of coloring in favor of the outside. Thus we were forced, though reluctantly, to dismiss all the experiments thus far made as having yielded doubtful results, excepting those made in the propagating-house, of which it will be necessary to speak further.*

How can we account for the results in this situation differing from those of the other rooms? At this time we were unable to find any good reason, the conditions appearing to be about the same. Subsequent experimentation, however, threw new light upon this vexed question. It will be necessary to state here what we trust will be evident to the mind of the reader later on; that the somewhat more striking results in this house must have been due to the fact that it was well stocked with flowering geraniums.

---

* My acknowledgments are due Mr. Menje for valuable assistance while conducting these experiments.

It became evident that in order to set at rest this important question, the conditions would have to be varied and further observations instituted. We now set to work to devise the necessary apparatus to carry on such experiments. Accordingly, we had made a glass case large enough to contain a dozen or more thrifty growing plants in pots. Its dimensions were as follows: Length, three and a half feet; width, two and a half feet; and height, two and a half feet. A portion of the top was left removable, so as to furnish an aperture through which the plants could be placed in the case and again taken out. This arrangement admitted the sunlight to the plants and confined their exhalations, while it would give the ozone, should any be generated, the best opportunity of acting upon the test-papers. In all of the remaining experiments in reference to the question of the generation of ozone by plant growth, I was greatly assisted by Dr. G. B. M. Miller, then my medical student. The apparatus was first placed in the bay-window of an occupied sitting-room facing east. The plants here received the sun's rays for at least six hours of the day. A dozen thrifty plants were placed in the case, which was then accurately closed by the removable piece of glass already spoken of, the test-papers having been moistened and tacked on the branches or stems of the plants. In the first series of experiments flowering plants were used, twelve in number, each bearing several flowers, and each presenting about four square feet of leaf-surface. They consisted of varieties of geraniums, fuchsias, begonias, hydrangeas, and petunias. Upon these plants eighteen observations were made of about four hours each, during the latter part of the month of May, 1883; weather mostly fair. For seven experiments the Schönbein showed "very slight" indications and one "slight," there being ten negative results. The guaiacum-papers gave more striking results, the change in the papers being "marked" for ten of the experiments, and, save one which was negative, "slight" for the remaining trials. Great care was taken to keep the plants experimented with in a healthy condition; they were also left in the pots in which they had been growing. There are two reasons which can be assigned why the results of these experiments were not very striking with the iodized starch test. First, our experiments were of too short duration; secondly, they were conducted in-doors, since the air of the case was originally the air of the room, and a portion at least of the ozone which might have been generated by the plants would have been decomposed by the impurities of the air in the case.

With a full knowledge of the unfavorable conditions under which these experiments were conducted, but encouraged by their moderate success, we resolved to make a trial of odoriferous flowering plants under the same conditions. Again our little floral chamber was filled with plants, consisting of seven rose-bushes, four carnation pinks, and six heliotropes. The duration of observations being about ten diurnal hours each; weather mostly clear, two days cloudy. With the Schönbein test there were "very slight" reactions, in most instances two "slight" and one well "marked," while the guaiacum-papers were "marked" in most cases, two being "slight." The number of experiments were eight. These experiments naturally suggested the idea that odorous flowering plants might be better ozone-generators than inodorous ones. During the time of the preceding serial experiments the external atmospheric conditions were very similar, the maximum temperature ranging from 85° to 88° Fahr. Repeated testing of the atmosphere of the room in which the case was situated gave no indication of the presence of ozone. The question now very naturally emerged, whether the colorations were due to ozone or to some of the substances which give the same reactions with these papers; hence, further investigation was necessary in order to exclude, if possible, these interfering conditions, before it could be claimed for plants that they were capable of emitting or converting the oxygen of the air into ozone. It was also deemed important to conduct future experiments out of doors, as, for reasons already given, it was expected more decided results would be obtained. The case was removed to the back yard, which lies to the eastward of the dwelling. Here the plants received the sunlight for at least eight hours of the daily experiments during clear weather. The yard was of good size. In the first series of experiments in this locality the plants last named were employed.

After observations for seven consecutive days of clear weather, the Schönbein paper gave "slight" reactions in four cases and "marked" reactions in three. The guaiacum-paper gave "slight" indications in three and "marked" in four experiments. Our readers will see that these experiments gave more marked results than those made within-doors. It was found, it may be

HOUSE-PLANTS AS SANITARY AGENTS. 127

stated, that the coloration of the Schönbein or iodized starch test was "slight" instead of "very slight" as in-doors, and in three cases actually "marked" against one "marked" result in the preceding series. The guaiacum tests were almost correspondingly more marked. It is quite probable that the more surprising results of the last series are not attributable solely to the change of location, but also in some degree to the fact that the individual experiments were of longer duration. A piece of red litmus suspended in the case during these experiments gave no indication of the presence of ammonia. Peroxide of hydrogen could not have been the reactionary agent, since that substance is decomposed at a temperature of 70° Fahr., while the temperature of the atmosphere within the case, this being carefully noted, was never found to be below 90° Fahr. These observations were made during the first week in June, 1883, the weather being very warm and the temperature of the air within the case being higher than that of the external air. Good reactions were, however, in later experiments, obtained when the temperature did not mark over 70° Fahr. That the reactions were not due to the nitrous oxides, perhaps the only remaining substance capable of producing like colorations of these test-papers, will appear evident hereafter.

We next proposed to give foliage plants having soft thin leaves a trial. For experimentation, seven asperdistei, one fern, and three dracænæ were chosen. These observations were conducted for seven consecutive days during the first week in September, 1883. The weather was extremely warm, the temperature of the air within the case varying from 85° to 100° Fahr. The sky was clear during four, and cloudy the remaining three days. The Schönbein test-paper gave throughout negative results, while the guaiacum gave one "very slight" reaction, the rest being negative also. Thus it would appear that foliage plants have not this power of generating ozone. The function must therefore reside with the flower, but of its nature we shall hereafter speak.

As our first experiments with inodorous flowering plants did not yield results striking enough to afford a basis for positive conclusions, we considered it desirable to apply the tests to them in the open air, which was done. Seventeen thrifty geraniums were employed. The temperature during these experiments was lower than during those made in-doors with inodorous plants. For six consecutive days, the experiments being of ten hours' duration each, the Schönbein gave one negative, two "slight" and three "marked" blue shades; the negative result occurred on a rainy day, during which there was no sunshine whatever. This would suggest the idea that sunlight, or at least good diffused light, is essential to the generation of ozone by plants, since our plants were protected from the rain by the glass. There are, as our readers are aware, other physiological phenomena carried on by plants which are largely dependent upon the power of the sun's rays, namely, assimilation and transpiration.

Upon those plants observations were continued during the second week of September, the results being about similar to those last noted; the Schönbein giving two "marked," one negative, on a rainy day, and the rest "slight" reactions. The guaiacum papers furnished two "marked" and the remainder "slight" colorations. As before intimated, nitrous oxides, when present in the air, change the color of these test-papers very much as ozone does. To exclude the possibility of the alteration in color being due to the nitrous oxides, we tested simultaneously the air on the outside of the case, and found that the papers in this situation gave only one "slight" reaction, and even though this occasional reaction on the exterior had been due to the presence of the nitrous oxides, they could not have caused the more striking and constant results obtained on the inside. Again, it is not at all likely that the plants generated nitrous oxides, which in turn might have changed the test-papers, for there is nothing in all vegetable physiology to support such an hypothesis.

Moreover, it is all the more improbable that nitrous oxides caused the above colorations, since they did not do so *when foliage plants were employed*.

We do not wish to say dogmatically that all the modifications in the test-papers were due to ozone, but from the numerous beautiful reactions obtained, and the systematic precautions taken to preclude the action of other substances known to answer to like tests, it will not be denied that this was the chief agent altering the papers. I was unable to discover the odor of ozone upon which Professor Leeds lays so much stress, but Mr. Miller thought he could detect its presence. It must be borne in mind that the amount of plant life within the case was probably too small to generate sufficient ozone to make it perceptible to the sense of smell.

In the light of the present experiments, there can scarcely be a doubt but a manifest relation does exist between vegetation and the ozonic condition of the atmosphere. And this, it will be conceded, is not the least hygienic influence possessed by plants. During fair weather all flowering vegetation is contributing ozone to the atmosphere. In this connection it should be noted that vegetation is largely blooming, that numerous field plants, the forest-trees as well as fruit-trees, put forth flowers, and that during this period they all add their quota of ozone to the surrounding medium. Again, not all blooming plants or trees produce their flowers at the same time of the season, and it thus happens that there are a certain proportion of different species flowering in turn from early spring till late in autumn, and hence the effect upon the atmosphere with reference to the amount of ozone they give to it must be pretty constant during the whole vegetative period wherever plant growth abounds. We here have another evidence of the fact that in His eternal wisdom the Author of nature has intrusted to plant life the task of maintaining the harmonious composition of the atmosphere.

From the results of the foregoing experiments two chief conclusions are to be deduced. First, that flowering plants in general possess the power to generate ozone, and odorous flowers in particular. Secondly, that foliage plants do not possess this function.

Later, a reinvestigation was undertaken with a view either of confirming or disproving the above deductions. Owing to the high significance which attaches to the question of the relation of plant growth to atmospheric ozone, as well as the fact that the true nature of the ozone-producing function in plants was still an unsettled problem, this course was deemed almost incumbent.

The second group of researches, which will be found to be not less interesting than the first, was conducted jointly with my gifted friend and pupil, Dr. George B. M. Miller. Partly because they are excellent in themselves, and partly because the results tend to demonstrate further a new truth which once definitely settled can be shown to have important relations to the public welfare, they will be, even at the risk of straining the indulgence of the reader, here reproduced.

The apparatus employed in the former experiments, namely, the glass casing, the same test-papers, etc., being likewise used in the present researches, a further description of them here would be a work of supererogation. In the present experiments the same terminology as in the former, namely, "marked," "slight," and "very slight," to denote the degree of blue coloration, was employed.

A dozen thrifty plants belonging to the species *Coleus Blumei*, not blooming, were first selected and placed within the glass case. The test-papers were moistened and suspended on the branches of the plants. After adjusting the removable part of our case, the latter was found to be pretty well filled, though not overstocked, with plant growth. For the purpose of detecting any alkaline substance, whose presence, it is said, will change the Schönbein and guaiacum papers in a manner indistinguishable from that produced by ozone, we suspended with the test-papers a piece of red litmus, with the results indicated in the following tables. The air on the exterior of the case was simultaneously tested for ozone. In a subsequent table, the results from the before-named specimens for seven consecutive days in the month of June, 1884, are, for the student's inspection, carefully recorded. With the Schönbein paper two "slight" reactions occurred, but since on the same days the red litmus was changed to a marked blue, there is a strong probability that these results were due to the presence of some alkaline substance. Thus, after repeated experiments, it would appear indubitable that it cannot be claimed for non-odorous foliage plants that they are ozone-generating. Though the guaiacum-paper gave "slight" results in three experiments which yielded no reactions with the litmus-paper, owing to the fact that this paper is materially affected by various atmospheric conditions, we did not much rely upon the results obtained from its employment. On the other hand, if proper precautionary measures be taken, the Schönbein is doubtless, as before mentioned, of all the tests for ozone the most reliable. These results are in exact accord with those previously recorded by one of us (*supra*).

We next experimented with odorless flowering plants, selecting ten of the species *Fuchsia globosa*, and ten periwinkles, species *Vinca rosea*, gaining rather meagre results (see *post*, p. 137). During the observations upon these plants, which were made during a period of seven days in the month of July, 1884, the temperature within the case ranged from 80° to 100° Fahr. Sufficient ozone was generated in four of the experiments to produce in the Schönbein paper one "marked" and three "very slight" reactions. The litmus gave no indication of the presence of ammonia. The average duration of the separate experiments was about ten hours. Although they do not rank as active ozone-generators, nevertheless they must, from the facts of the case, be looked upon as in a slight degree sharing this important function. This decision also coincides with what one of us had previously demonstrated by experiments.

A trial of odorous flowering plants was now made, selecting for this purpose seven roses and seven species of *Lilium longiflorum*. After carefully enclosing them within the case, the atmosphere of the latter was tested, and simultaneously the air outside, with striking results. From the Schönbein paper within the case we obtained, out of a total of eight experiments of about nine hours each duration, five "marked" and one "slight" reaction, while in the open air this paper gave us one "marked," one "slight," and two "very slight" results. During these experiments the temperature of the air in the case ranged from 80° to 100° Fahr.; weather for the most part clear.

The important conclusion arrived at in the previous papers,—namely, that odorous flowering plants are active and energetic ozone-producers,—it will be clear, receives from present researches entire confirmation.

This function having been shown to be carried on by odorous flowers, it occurred to us to make a trial of plants whose leaves emit odors, but are destitute of flowers. Blooming geraniums having been experimented with while making previous researches into the same subject, and having found them to be capable of generating ozone, it was determined to employ a number of specimens belonging to the genus Pelargonium *not in bloom*, with a view of ascertaining whether the reactions obtained with this species were due to the presence of the flower alone or whether, in whole or part, to the slightly odorous principles emitted from the leaves of the plants. To our astonishment, slight reactions were secured. The number of experiments with these plants was twelve, and the average duration of them about ten hours. Although there were but three "very slight" reactions, one "slight," and one "marked," with the Schönbein obtained in twelve observations made, this is not such a bad showing when it is recollected that four of the tests giving no indications of ozone were made on rainy days, it having been shown in the previous researches that sunlight, or at least good diffused light, is an essential condition to the generation of ozone by plants.

Upon this point, however, the evidence afforded by these experiments upon the foliage of the geraniums alone is too slender on which to base positive conclusions, and hence we deemed it desirable to make further observations by testing foliage possessing marked perfume. To aid in clearing up this subject, we next resolved to test pine foliage, which possesses the well-known terebinthinate odor, and in the results obtained we were not disappointed. Seven branches taken from the species *Pinus strobus* were introduced into the case in the upright position, and the same tests were applied to them as in the experiments on growing plants. The results for five experiments of about nine and one-half hours each were admirable. The Schönbein paper returned three "marked" reactions, one "slight," and one "negative" on the fifth day. After three days the pine branches turned brown and the leaves rapidly dropped off, facts which doubtless account for the negative results after the fourth experiment. It should be noted that we continued to test these branches on the sixth and seventh days respectively, and with negative results in both of the latter instances. We were, however, encouraged by the success attending the three first experiments, and resolved to make another trial of pine branches. Accordingly we again selected a half-dozen pines, which moderately filled our floral chamber, and allowed them to remain only until they began to show a change in color, which change occurred at the end of the third experiment. For three successive experiments with the Schönbein "marked" results were realized. The red litmus, neither during these nor the foregoing experiments with the pine branches, showed any change of color. We also made a serial of four daily experiments with branches taken from the Norway spruce (*Abies Canadensis*), with really happy results, the Schönbein giving us three " marked" tints, and one " slight." We unfortunately were unable at this time to obtain more foliage plants of the same character, and thus our investigations were brought to an end. Although a greater number of experiments upon this point could have been desired, when on the one hand it is recollected how great the difficulties connected with the making of such tests, and on the other the brilliant and unbroken success made with pine foliage, it will be readily conceded that these results, which were far from being expected, furnish abundant evidence of the ability on the part of the odorous principles evolved from the pine foliage to produce ozone.

From the present, together with the investigations previously detailed, we are at present writing justified in formulating the following conclusions:

First. That flowering plants, including odorous and inodorous, generate ozone, or convert the oxygen of the atmosphere into this substance, the former, however, much more actively than the latter.

Secondly. That so far as tested, scented foliage does possess the power to produce ozone, and in the case of pine or hemlock foliage to a marked degree.

Thirdly. That inasmuch as no reactions occurred on rainy days, it is highly probable that the function demands the influence of the sun's rays, or at least good diffused light. In comparing the present with the conclusions previously deduced, it will be seen that they differ only in so far as relates to foliage plants, those pertaining to flowering vegetation being perfectly concordant.

The following tabular record of our results has been compiled, for the definite purpose of showing that the above deductions rest solely upon carefully-conducted experiments; each series is preceded by the names of the plants and the number employed.

HOUSE-PLANTS AS SANITARY AGENTS.

Experiments with a dozen thrifty species of Coleus Blumei, not blooming.

Experiment.	Schönbein.	Guaiacum.	Schönbein. In open air.	Litmus (red).	Time.	State of Weather.
					Hours.	
I.	Negative.	Negative.	Negative.	Negative.	8	Clear.
II.	"	"	....	"	8	"
III.	Slight.	Marked.	Marked.	Blue.	11	"
IV.	Negative.	Slight.	Negative.	Negative.	9	"
V.	"	Very slight.	Marked.	"	9	"
VI.	"	"	Negative.	"	10	"
VII.	Slight.	Marked.	Slight.	Blue.	8	"

Experiments with ten plants of the species Fuchsia globosa, and ten Periwinkles, species Vinca rosea.

Experiment.	Schönbein.	Guaiacum.	Schönbein. In open air.	Litmus (red).	Time.	State of Weather.
					Hours.	
I.	Marked.	Marked.	Negative.	Negative.	10	Clear.
II.	Negative.	"	Marked.	"	9	"
III.	"	Negative.	Negative.	"	10	"
IV.	Very slight.	Slight.	Slight.	"	13	"
V.	"	Negative.	"	"	9	"
VI.	"	Slight.	Marked.	"	9	"
VII.	Negative.	"	"	"	10	"

Experiments with seven Roses and seven specimens Lilium longiflorum.

Experiment.	Schönbein.	Guaiacum.	Schönbein. In open air.	Litmus (red).	Time.	State of Weather.
					Hours.	
I.	Negative.	Marked.	Negative.	Blue.	8	Clear.
II.	Marked.	"	"	Negative.	9	"
III.	Negative.	Negative.	"	"	9	Partly cloudy.
IV.	Slight.	Marked.	Marked.	"	8	Clear.
V.	Marked.	"	Slight.	"	10	"
VI.	"	"	Very slight.	"	10	"
VII.	"	"	"	"	11	"
VIII.	"	"	Negative.	"	10½	"

Experiments with a dozen species of Pelargonium, not in bloom.

Experiment	Schönbein.	Guaiacum.	Schönbein. In open air.	Litmus (red).	Time.	State of Weather.
					Hours.	
I.	Very slight.	Slight.	Marked.	Negative.	10	Clear.
II.	Negative.	Negative.	"	"	10	"
III.	"	"	"	"	10	"
IV.	"	"	Negative.	"	10	Rainy.
V.	Very slight.	Very slight.	"	"	10	Clear.
VI.	Negative.	Slight.	"	"	9	"
VII.	Very slight.	"	Marked.	"	9	Partly cloudy.
VIII.	Negative.	Negative.	Negative.	"	10	Rainy.
IX.	"	Marked.	Marked.	"	11	Clear.
X.	Marked.	Slight.	Slight.	"	10	"
XI.	Slight.	"	Negative.	"	9	Cloudy.
XII.	Negative.	Negative.	"	"	10	Rainy.

Experiments with seven branches from the species Pinus strobus.

Experiment	Schönbein.	Guaiacum.	Schönbein. In open air.	Litmus (red).	Time.	State of Weather.
					Hours.	
I.	Marked.	Slight.	Very slight.	Negative.	9	Clear.
II.	"	Marked.	Slight.	"	10	"
III.	"	"	"	"	9	"
IV.	Slight.	Slight.	Marked.	"	10	"
V.	Negative.	Negative.	"	"	9	"

Experiments with a half-dozen branches of the Pinus strobus.

Experiment	Schönbein.	Guaiacum.	Schönbein. In open air.	Litmus (red).	Time.	State of Weather.
					Hours.	
I.	Marked.	Marked.	Marked.	Negative.	9	Clear.
II.	"	Slight.	Negative.	"	10	Clear, partly cloudy.
III.	"	"	Slight.	"	10	Clear.

Experiments with branches from the Norway Spruce (Abies Canadensis).

Experiment.	Schönbein.	Guaiacum.	Schönbein. In open air.	Litmus (red).	Time.	State of Weather.
					Hours	
I.	Marked.	Marked.	Slight.	Negative.	12	Clear.
II.	"	Slight.	Negative.	"	10	"
III.	Slight.	Marked.	"	"	10	"
IV.	Marked.	Slight.	Marked.	"	9	"

What is the nature of this ozone-producing process? may be pertinently asked.

From present premises, it appears evident that the odoriferous principle emitted, whether from flower or foliage, is in some way chiefly concerned in its formation. It is true we are unable in this manner to account for its production by odorless flowers, unless, as many contend, we grant that all blossoms are either bedecked with or somewhere in their loose cellular tissue contain scented nectar, which in many so-called inodorous flowers may not be sufficiently marked to be perceived by the organ of smell. It is a fact well established that, wherever fertilization is accomplished by insects, so-called nectaries are somewhere to be found in the flowers. These organs are by Sachs ("Text-Book of Botany," p. 510) briefly described as follows: "The nectaries are often nothing but glandular portions of tissue in the axial or foliar parts of the flower; very often they project in the form of cushions of more delicate tissue, or take the form of stalked or sessile protuberances; or whole foliar structures of the perianth of the andrœcium or even of the gynœcium, are transformed into peculiar structures for the secretion and accommodation of the nectar."

The proportion of plants in which pollination is effected by insects is certainly very great, and when we take into account those cases in which cross fertilization results from the same agency, this proportion becomes much greater.

Whether it can with justice be claimed for all inodorous flowers that they contain a greater or lesser number of nectaries, we are not prepared to state; but certain it is, that numerous flowers which are classed as being without fragrance, or any other odors, such as the geranium, the passion flower, and others, are visited by insects, and these must therefore contain glandular tissues filled with an alluring secretion. Here the question naturally arises, Are there not flowers, not visited by insects, which flowers possess these glandular organs?

Our view that the fragrant emanations from flowers, as well as all the odorous substances emitted from plants, stand in close relation to the ozone-producing function in plants, receives further confirmatory proof in the pretty generally accepted chemical fact that the volatile perfumes which are found upon the market have the power to produce or to convert the oxygen of the atmosphere into ozone.

It is gratifying to note that soon after the publication of our investigations into this subject there fell under our notice a curt statement coming from high authority, claiming for an Italian professor the discovery of the fact that vegetable perfumes convert the oxygen of the air into ozone. According to this observer, whose name does not appear, the flowers of the narcissus, hyacinth, mignonette, and lily of the valley develop ozone in closed vessels. Flowers destitute of perfumes did not develop it, and those having but slight perfumes developed it in small quantities. No observations by this gentleman looking to the solution of the ozonizing influence residing in the exhalations from foliar organs or pines have been recorded. Some essences, and among them those of the cherry, laurel, clover, lavender, mint, juniper, lemon, fennel, and bergamot, develop this substance in great abundance, while others, such as the anise, nutmeg, and thyme, generate it less rapidly.

So far, then, as appertains to the flowering species, these results do not differ materially from our own, except in the particular which attributes to inodorous flowers the power to form a slight amount of this substance. The harmony of this remarkable concurrence of results, and the conclusions of each being reached independently of the other, still more forcibly attest the exactness of our hypothesis already adduced. At all events the purifying and healthful influence upon our atmosphere of the various vegetable perfumes, either from flower or foliage, seems now to be completely established.

A certain proportion of ozone in the atmosphere doubtless is essential to prevent it from becoming too greatly polluted for human respiration by organic matter and by the products of decomposition, particularly azotized substances, which are known to be a fruitful cause of disease. Not only so, but the latter are by some believed to serve as carriers for the germs of epidemic diseases.

Indeed, that ozone, in general terms, through its power to combine chemically with pernicious organic impurities, constitutes nature's chief means of purifying our atmosphere, which impurities cause, as medical authorities well know, manifold forms of suffering, rendering the air unfit for purposes of breathing, is no longer a mere probability, but rather a demonstrated fact. This point is confirmed by Professor Kedzie of the University of Michigan, who tells us that he regards ozone as the most energetic of the constituents of the atmosphere. "Its presence or absence must have a *controlling influence over the vital powers*, and when we consider that this material is present in such variable amount in a medium which surrounds us every moment of our lives, and whose action pauses not for matin or for vesper, at noon of day or noon of night, it seems to me that no one can deny that its influence on human health must be most significant."

Of the sanitary value of ozone in the air, that high authority, Professor Max von Pettenkofer (*loc. cit.*), says, "It is the constant purifier of the atmosphere from all organic matter which passes into it and might accumulate. The air would have been long ago filled with the vapors of decomposition if it were not for ozone, which oxidizes all that is oxidizable if only time be allowed for it, and not too much is expected at once."

How long it would be possible for animal life to exist were the atmospheric ozone to be suddenly annihilated, cannot be computed, but that existence would sooner or later become impossible on account of noxious substances which would accumulate in the air and which it is the office of ozone to destroy, cannot, we think, be reasonably doubted. How infinitely wise and beneficent, then, is the Author of all nature in placing beside these destroying elements a most salutary remedial measure, namely, plants and flowers acting as natural and effective ozone-generators!

From the facts brought out by the results of scientific research, it is clearly seen that the cultivation of blooming as well as non-blooming plants giving off perfumes in marshy localities and all other places in which the air is greatly polluted by the products of decaying organic material cannot be, on account of the great energy which ozone manifests to destroy these injurious elements, too strongly recommended. It is equally clear and not less important for our readers to observe how decidedly beneficial scented foliage and flowering plants must become in the presence of all public gatherings; so that the practice, which is and has been flourishing, of beautifying by means of these graceful objects of nature on occasions of even the least public significance, has a twofold action, of which the sanitary influence is not the least valuable.

Thus they would be of special value in the theatre, in the crowded lecture-hall, the church, and so on. Of course, in order to be effective when used under these conditions, it is important that they should be introduced at least twenty-four hours before their effects would be required.

But the most interesting practical phase of the agreeable results of our researches is their application to the question of cultivation of house-plants. As before mentioned, ozone is not detectable in living-rooms. It will be recollected by the reader that plants during clear weather generate ozone when kept in-doors. Reasoning from the effects of a dozen thrifty plants in a case of the dimensions of the one employed in our experiments, it can scarcely be doubted that a sufficient number of flowering varieties to stock a living- or sleeping-apartment would, during fair weather, generate enough ozone to be of decided sanitary value. For in this connection it should be further remarked that we rarely find in the outer air more than a small quantity, which yet appears to be adequate to maintain it in a salubrious condition.

In general terms, the air of our dwellings is truly abominable, being charged with deleterious substances which serve admirably as a culture-fluid for the various disease-producing germs.

These injurious materials incessantly pervading the house air arise from various more or less distinctive sources. Some of these it is well briefly to consider, if the reader wishes to obtain a good idea as to the extent of noxious substances to which he is constantly exposed. We have first to mention human respiration, which slowly but constantly contaminates the air of the home, and more particularly if proper ventilation be not observed. We have previously spoken of the pernicious influences of an excess of carbon dioxide in the air of the living-room attributable to this same phenomenon, but an equally important factor is the organic matter given off in respiration. A minor evil resulting from imperfect ventilation of closed rooms is the consequent accumulation of irritant matter, such as particles of coal, clothing, etc., which are suspended in the atmosphere and do considerable mischief by invading the air-passages. Another source of contamination, and one deserving our most attentive study, because truly fearful in its effects, is escaping sewer gas. A perfect system of drainage would, it is obvious, prevent the possibility of such an accident, but unfortunately, as the result of the proverbial carelessness and incompetency of the generality of plumbers, a contrary state of things usually exists, and sewer air is allowed to pass almost unchecked into our dwellings. Its composition, though extremely variable, is as a rule dangerous. The famous Sanitarian Parkes ("Manual of Practical Hygiene," vol. i. p. 128) tells us that the gases entering into sewer air, of which the most common are carbon dioxide, nitrogen, and frequently ammonium sulphide and hydrogen sulphide, are in comparison with the organic fetid matters of far less significance. In sewer air, as some writers likewise point out, fungi grow rapidly, while meat and milk when exposed to it soon taint.

Now, although their true nature has not been as yet accurately determined, that the morbific agents producing diphtheria, scarlet fever, typhoid fever, are in many instances traceable to the invasion into our dwellings of sewer air, has by numerous medical writers been established fully.

The view that troublesome diarrhœa and dysentery are frequently caused by sewer emanations is also no longer problematical.

Again, the numerous forms of fungi and living ferments (bacteria) found in the external atmosphere naturally gain entrance to our living-chambers, and these here find sadly too often a suitable nidus for their propagation and development. These are generally acknowledged to be the cause of the class of diseases known as zymotic. In this connection it should be noted that there are purifying influences at work in the open air, which influences do not in any degree come into play within-doors, notably wind and rain. Now, while some of the contaminating influences brought forward are not in constant operation, others practically are, namely, human respiration, imperfect ventilation, and the impurities derived from the exterior; hence the fact remains that the air of the home is quite generally positively pernicious in its effects upon human health. So long as this state of things exists, no vigorous argument is necessary to show the importance of placing the house under more favorable hygienic influences.

Than to attend to these matters there is nothing more needful to keep the body in a prime, healthy condition. To the end of attaining this happy result it is not our purpose to underrate the value of the ordinary sanitary measures; on the contrary, we cannot too strongly emphasize the importance of cleanliness and proper ventilation; but in view of the fact that plants, as demonstrated by our investigations, possess the power to produce ozone, which, on its part, is powerful to destroy the organic ingredients, and possibly even the disease-germs, —of all infectious elements the most perilous,—our readers doubtless will be almost unanimously in agreement with us in assigning to house-plants, for the above reasons alone, a prominent place as health-giving agents. Owing, however, to our present limited knowledge concerning the exact quantity of ozone poured into the air by plant growth, and to the fact that much time is required for ozone to effect its work of purification, let it be distinctly understood that in our present position to claim for this ozonizing function in plants, the power under ordinary circumstances *to remove from the air all poisonous substances* would be irrational, but on the other side there can be little doubt that a proper ratio of flowering plants grown within-doors would in this direction be decidedly efficacious. Next to transpiration, then, in point of hygienic import, we must rank this freshly-discovered process of nature. For the purpose of protecting our homes from the influence of the poisonous materials usually contained in the external atmosphere, the cultivation of foliage and flowering plants endowed with fragrance on the exterior, but in close proximity to the house, might be suggested. In the bed-chamber, it may be confidently asserted, plants would correct the ill effects of the organic exhalations of the slumbering household. To their peculiarly happy effect in the sick-chamber we shall hereafter allude. Finally, it is to be noted that whenever atmospheric impurities are likely to endanger human health, then house-plants should, without the slightest fear of being hostile in themselves, be introduced.

There is a peculiarly happy and pleasing aspect of our subject presented in what are commonly known as the moral influences of plants and flowers. While this influence has never been, and is not now, open to dispute, few have perhaps appreciated its real significance. In this connection, then, are to be noted especially the refining and softening influences upon human mind and character of the practice of floriculture,—a fact well worthy of permanent preservation. As agents to delight the mind, to afford rest by agreeably entertaining the mind, to divert the attention and to relieve ennui, they cannot be too heartily advocated. By the happy observation for which we believe the *London Medical Record* of recent date is responsible, namely, that plants and flowers are valuable as *delassement* for the weak and weary, the same idea is beautifully expressed. Who has not felt in an especial degree the pleasure at witnessing the gorgeous beauty of some chamber handsomely decorated with ornamental plants, or it may be the floral adornments of the well-laden table of some hospitable host, groaning under the most palatable luxuries of the season? It has also been pointed out that the presence of plants and flowers in the family circle gives a feeling of companionship, and thus they might not infrequently, on this ground alone, serve to brighten the lonely hours of the thrifty housewife. To see that subtle thinker and eminent writer upon sanitary matters, Professor Max von Pettenkofer, with whom our readers have already been made familiar, taking the same view, is exceedingly gratifying. He continues, " I consider flowers in a room, for all to whom they give pleasure, to be one of the enjoyments of life, like condiments in food." Our readers will doubtless, in view of these facts, and more particularly as the superstitious fancies of former times no longer hold sway, be ready to commit themselves to the idea that there are most excellent reasons for ushering the treasures of the greenhouse into our living-rooms for the benefit they confer in ministering to our æsthetic taste and gratifying our senses.

To behold a living-chamber laden with flowering

and leaf plants graceful in themselves, and evincing in their arrangement something of the gardener's art, has always been cherished as one of the rarest pleasures of our lives. But how transcendently grand and resplendent the mental impression produced by the beautiful landscape in spring-time, presenting as far as the eye can reach its beautiful carpets of green verdure, marked here and there either by ornamental shrubbery or solitary trees, or it may be by the sombre forest in the distance, whose colossal oaks seemingly cleave the very skies! By the side of this picture we behold the autumn foliage, enriched by its varied and delicately-tinted colors, forming another whose inimitable grace and grandeur gives evidence of being of divine conception and execution. Surely such observations alone sufficiently prove that to vegetation must be accorded the proud distinction of lending both to spring and autumn their most distinctive charms. It is a matter for little surprise, then, that man should become a votary at the shrine of our beautiful floral empire.

On reviewing briefly the preceding discussion of the sanitary relations of plants and flowers, we observe them to be thrice illustrious: as perfect and brilliant atomizers of aqueous vapors, as natural ozone-producers, and as moral agencies. Having endeavored to point out the true significance of these various plant functions each in detail, we would briefly recapitulate a few points of chiefest practical importance, but we wish more particularly to attempt to indicate the proper ratio of plant-growth for sanitary uses. Our readers will recall the rate at which soft thin foliage exhales aqueous vapor, namely, one and a quarter ounces *per diem* for each square foot of leaf-surface,—a ratio which, when we take into account the vast extent of leaf-surface exposed by even a small collection of plants, becomes almost startling in its proportions. It will be remembered that by virtue of their power to increase the atmospheric moisture they maintain a proper standard of humidity of the air of living-rooms. But equal to this in practical import there is the fact of the plant moisture being distilled with greater uniformity of rate than from other sources,—a consideration, it will be recollected, possessing inestimable hygienic advantages. Short of this it is perhaps most noteworthy to recount on the one hand the manifold forms of ill consequences arising from the employment of the dry-air furnace as a method of heating, and on the other the efficient service of living plants as reparatory measures.

Regarding the ability of plants to develop ozone, little indeed remains to be added. In common with transpiration, the work of forming ozone is largely accomplished by the influence of the solar rays. In order to facilitate a practical application of the data gained by our experimental exploration of this phenomenon, it is well to keep in remembrance those plants which are most active and those least so, as ozone-generators; among the former are to be noted scented foliage and flowers, the latter embracing chiefly inodorous flowers, while inodorous foliage is powerless to engender ozone. The last named are not, however, to be discarded in the selection of plants for in-door cultivation, since there are other important hygienic advantages to be derived from their presence. Not to speak of the pleasing effects produced by their natural beauty, they can boast among their number some good transpirers of aqueous vapor. In the use of plants for hygienic purposes we have elsewhere (see "Hygienic and Therapeutic Relation of Plants," *Philadelphia Medical Times*, May 8, 1880) prepared a formula as follows: given a room twenty feet long, twelve feet wide, and ceiling twelve feet high, warmed by dry air, a dozen thrifty plants with soft thin leaves and a leaf-surface of six square feet each would, if well watered, and so situated as to receive the direct rays of the sun (preferably the morning sun) for at least several hours, raise the proportion of aqueous vapor to about the health standard. It is to be remarked here that this formula was framed prior to our researches into the ozone-producing function on the part of growing plants. Moreover, these later investigations have shown clearly that in order to develop sufficient ozone to be of service in keeping up an agreeable state of purity of our atmosphere, it is necessary to increase the above proportion of flowers. More recently we have, with proper regard to this fact, endeavored to modify carefully the form above prescribed, as follows: given a room twenty feet long, twelve feet wide, and ceiling twelve feet high, warmed by dry air, not less than twenty thrifty growing plants, if possible flower-bearing and varieties giving off odors,—having soft thin leaves and a leaf-surface of six square feet each,—would be, if properly watered, and situated so as to receive the direct rays of the sun, an appropriate adjustment.

To obtain the very best results, both the rooms occupied during the day and the sleeping-apartments should contain plants. But for obvious reasons, which need not detain us here, the bed-chamber would in general require a lesser proportion. In summer, plants should, whenever opportunity is not wanting, be cultivated in the open air as well. Indeed, these precious and natural health-giving objects should properly be regarded as those among our associates whose constant companionship would at all times return the greatest blessings. Among the numerous forms of diversion at our command, the practice of floriculture, which is neither difficult nor costly, should be held to be one of the foremost. Than the intimate association of certain of the principal plant-functions with the laws of hygiene, nothing more beautifully or more forcibly attests the infinite wisdom and kind beneficence of the Author of our Universe toward His dependent subjects. And to behold important sanitary influences residing in mysterious physiological functions of living vegetation can scarcely fail to inspire all with admiration and reverence for His enactment of natural laws which contribute so largely to the health and comfort of mankind.

CHAPTER VI.

House-plants as sanitary agents in the sick-room—Their effect to prevent the transmission of communicable diseases—Their value in acute febrile diseases and especially during the convalescence from the latter—Hygienic importance of the Solarium in hospitals—House-plants especially valuable in the chambers of chronic invalids—Their therapeutic application in functional nervous disorders—In inflammation of the throat—In true croup—In acute and chronic bronchitis and laryngitis—Description of different forms of chronic bronchitis—Advantages of growing plants in their treatment—Proportion of plants required—The value of living plants as preventives of bronchitis.

FROM what in the previous chapter has been stated concerning the sanitary purposes to which growing plants are subservient, the professional reader, at any rate, will not experience great surprise at hearing the announcement of the proposition that they must be in the sick-room of signal value both as sanitary and therapeutic agencies. The weight of the testimony gathered from our own researches is in the highest degree favorable to this assumption. Again, if, as has been before shown, constant companionship with floral life tends to preserve good health to the healthy individual, it is natural to expect them to be efficient as agents of prevention in different forms of disease. But there is, happily, sufficient evidence at hand of a practical kind to establish this view completely. Though to attempt to draw a strict line of distinction between their hygienic and therapeutic application would be an unnecessary refinement of terms, it is my purpose, for the sake of convenience as well as a desire to render the discussion easily comprehensible, to consider three subdivisions of the present branch of the subject, successively.

I. The sanitary uses of house-plants in the sick-chamber.

II. Their therapeutic application in sundry affections with particular regard to affections of the mucous membranes of the air-passages.

III. Their power to prevent, and their value in confirmed, phthisis.

In speaking of the sanitary advantages of plants in the sick-room, we refer chiefly to their usage in accordance with the formula previously laid down for hygienic purposes in health, with perhaps slight variations, which will be noted in special indications. Of course, under these circumstances it is not to be expected either to forestall any particular disease or to modify to any extent its course, but there can be no doubt whatever that in numerous diseases the ozone-producing and transpiring properties of plants, together with their æsthetic influences, would greatly contribute to the physical comfort and mental gratification of the patient. Doubtless the larger proportion of the zymotic and inflammatory diseases (except in the case of acute rheumatism, the reasons for which will hereafter appear), or at all events those which by reason of their great virulence are known to victimize the largest percentage of subjects, such as typhoid fever, diphtheria, scarlet fever, etc., are by the best mycologists supposed to be caused by a specific germ, which, though in most cases unknown, is no doubt peculiar to each. Now, it is quite probable that the ozone developed by a good ratio of flowering plants, such as before indicated, would be adequate to clarify to a great extent the air of the invalid's chamber by destroying some of the disease-producing germs, or, if this in the present condition of our knowledge be claiming too much for the action of ozone, it certainly will not appear extravagant to maintain for this energetic body the power to consume by oxidation a variety of organic atmospheric impurities which would otherwise serve as carriers or transmitters of the specific agencies causing disease. Obviously, the danger of disseminating any of the contagious and infectious diseases might in this manner be greatly diminished. The organic exhalations from the skin and lungs of the patient—substances which, as pointed out in the previous chapter, are highly injurious in their effects, being greatly prone to decomposition—would also be attacked and annihilated by the ozone developed by the plants. The acute febrile disorders furnish a good opportunity for the moist vapors emitted to produce a truly delightful effect in soothing and cooling the restless, feverish frame of the patient. In all instances in which the mucous membrane of the pharynx or air-passages is the seat of catarrhal inflammation, or even graver changes, a somewhat larger ratio than above set down would, by continuous atomization of the parts, be of superior advantage. But in the latter category of cases we will hereafter presume to rank growing plants as therapeutic agencies. If it be true that a deeply implanted love for plants and flowers appears to be indigenous to the human heart, and that most persons are fond of having them in their living-apartments, how much greater the pleasure and gratification they would give to persons who are confined to a sick-bed! To the drooping spirits from which the majority of patients, independently of the character of illness, suffer, the fascinating and enheartening influence of house-plants is unquestionable.

Doubtless, during the period of convalescence from any of the acute diseases referred to, plants would prove their virtues to be peculiarly advantageous. Unless aided by the physician's art, full recovery would ofttimes be not only lengthily drawn out, but also in some cases unattainable. Now, whilst it is not my wish to uphold the use of plants to the damage of all the other measures which the medical profession has come to regard as of value to convalescents, it is *my desire* to sanction their use as aids to such medical measures with a most earnest endorsement. And this for good reasons. It is not irrational to aver that an atmosphere changed and rendered purer by growing plants would be more agreeable as well as more highly invigorating than otherwise. The singularly happy influence of good pure balmy air to promote sleep, to assist the appetite and digestion, is well known to the medical practitioner. The efficacy of plants in hastening the progress of recovery would be greatly enhanced by the admission of an abundance of sunlight, which in itself is accepted to be of great value on the one hand, and is, as the reader will recollect, the great agent in provoking both the formation of ozone and transpiration. Here again the members of the floral household, on account of their well-known power to gladden and to cheer, would, by the convalescing patients, be profoundly cherished. In beginning to take essential exercise, his first ramble should be among his plants, whether grown in-doors or out. To confirm this dictum concerning the hygienic benefits to be derived from house-plants, I purpose quoting from the writings upon this point of Dr. Pilcher a statement which sets forth the method adopted in a leading American hospital. "On the upper floor of the magnificent New York Hospital," says this writer, "is its *Solarium*, a large room with glass roof, where, among flowers and profuse foliage and murmuring fountains and genial sunshine, convalescent patients pass the hours of the day and hasten their returning strength." At the Hospital of the Protestant Episcopal Church at Philadelphia, the windows of the various wards as well as those of the large corridors contain plants, mainly flowering geraniums.

The vast assemblage of demonstrated facts furnishing positive proof of their sanitary advantages under proper regulation, leave no room for doubting that a general adoption of the practice in our hospitals where acute and chronic cases of illness are received for treatment, would, in the shape of solid benefit to the suffering occupants, return a handsome income on the slight outlay occasioned by their introduction. But in order to obtain the very best results, every hospital should afford a special apartment of good size,—dimensions not less than twenty by forty feet,—admitting an abundance of sunlight, and it should be thoroughly equipped by properly selected plants, the rules for which will be found to be fully stated in the chapter treating of Practical Floriculture, or in other words, if practicable, such a pleasant refuge as described to be practically exemplified in the New York Hospital should be universally imitated.

Except in a few special instances to be hereafter alluded to, converting the sick-room into a sanitarium by means of house-plants would be particularly desirable in chronic forms of disease necessitating confinement of the patient either to his room or to bed for long periods together. That good air is, in the event of every chronic invalid whose constant habitation is a single apartment, a paramount necessity no one can reasonably dispute. In these contingencies, dry furnace heat, owing to its long-continued action, produces exceedingly baneful consequences. So far as pertains to the results of furnace heat upon persons in good health, enough attention has previously been bestowed, while these ill effects in conditions of disease, it remains to be said, are expressed in a much more aggravated form, thus conducing greatly to the patient's discomfort, with rare exceptions. Since, therefore, as ordinarily met with, the air of the chronic invalid's abode is far from what it should be, ought we not to greet and to receive plants into these relations, for their remarkable meteorological effects, as among the most welcome of visitors? Furthermore, in none other more than in cases of a chronic nature could plants exhibit the power they possess to influence the mind and to attend to the gratification of the senses. Not alone the friends of the patient of this sort, but the attending physician as well, is aware how great the difficulty in perhaps all save the rarest circumstances, to guard them against growing dispirited and disheartened; and yet to keep them buoyant and cheerful is universally regarded as of high importance if the medicinal or other measures instituted are to be really efficacious. Who, in view of all the foregoing facts, could estimate the æsthetic value of plants and flowers to this large and varied class of sufferers, the mere enumeration of which would demand a separate chapter? Their potency to dispel gloom and to relieve measurably the tedium of life, are facts which alone furnish sufficient justification for their cultivation in these quarters.

Those diseased conditions in whose treatment plants deserve to be classed as therapeutic means will next be considered. House-plants have a noteworthy sphere of usefulness in certain nervous disorders of the functional class. Prominently among them stand to be mentioned melancholia and chlorosis, in diseases of the mind proper and in other allied conditions, such as excessive grief, ennui, and so on, where it is essential to divert the mind or to relieve tension. Than the pleasing occupation of studying and caring for plants, nothing in these cases is more productive of good results. Owing to the well-known fact that medicinal measures frequently are of little or no avail, and seeing that plants improve the wholesome qualities of the atmosphere of an inclosed space, they might in the above complaints form the chief, if not the sole reliance.

Certain maladies, it is well established, are greatly benefited by an atmosphere containing a higher degree of saturation than is called for by the ordinary health standard (or seven-eighths of what the air can contain at a given temperature, *supra*). To meet the demand in such ailments it is simply necessary to increase to the extent of twice, or perhaps in special instances thrice, the number of plants insisted upon for sanitary objects. As will be presently seen, those conditions to which plants are applicable are greatly diversified, and it would appear to be fair to assume that the amount of plant life should be equally varied, but such changes in the previous formula, and such only, will be made as seem to be coercive.

Reasoning both from adequate data gained by our investigations and from some amount of practical experience, it is mainly in chronic forms of disease, and particularly those affecting the air-passages, that we are to expect to derive the best results from such a measure as stocking the sick-room with growing vegetation. In this class of diseases, it will be remembered, dry heat is most harmful. Furthermore, in some acute diseases whose pathological lesions involve the respiratory tract as well as the pharynx, plants would prove themselves to be not much less efficient. To illustrate: every disease in which the throat is the seat of an inflammation, be this occasioned by taking cold, scarlet fever, diphtheria, or what it may, the plant-vapors diffused throughout the air of the room in a proper amount would, by moistening continually the parts through the act of respiration, produce a cooling and assuaging action, thus tending to diminish, to some extent at least, the severity of the local inflammatory action, and notably assist other measures in appeasing the victim's sufferings. When diseases of this class assume a pronounced type, which frequently occurs in scarlatina and diphtheria, the bodily temperature rises until the clinical thermometer registers anywhere from 100° to 105° Fahr., and remains so for days at a period. This likewise occurs in the so-called continued fevers, such as typhoid, typhus, and remittent fevers, with equal frequency. One of the results of this high temperature, which is due to the active febrile movement operating through the nervous centres, is to produce restlessness or even active delirium. Now, one of the effects of a more or less humid plant air, if the atmospheric temperature be maintained at from 65° to 70° Fahr., upon the fever patient is to allay the excessive heat of skin over exposed portions of the body, as well as to aid in allaying nervous excitement, thus eminently favoring his repose. But that some share of the credit in the production of this favorable influence is due to the ozone developed and emitted must be held to be tolerably certain, since from the writings of Eyseline (*Arch. de Neurol.*), who has made a sufficient number of observations in hospital practice to enable him to speak positively, it would appear to be fully proved that its effects upon the human race are sedative and hypnotic. If future observation in this new and interesting field tend to confirm completely the conclusions of this observer, then it is seen that the range of therapeutic applicability of house-plants would thereby be greatly widened. To show still further the felicitous influence of house-plants upon the nervous system, the author craves the kind reader's permission to place on record an illustrative case in point which quite recently came to his notice. A lady little short of middle life had been for a period of many months suffering from a condition of neurosis. Without stopping to describe all the ill-defined symptoms rendering her life miserable, it should be specially pointed out that she declared the most wearying concomitant in her case was sleeplessness. After making a trial of various nervines with no permanent relief, and having previously informed herself as to the promising sanitary merits of growing plants, she optionally concluded to supply well her bed-chamber with blooming plants, which was done without delay. The result was most gratifying. She soon expressed herself as feeling better and as being less troubled with sleeplessness.

Than the disease diversely called "membranous laryngitis," "true croup," "pseudo-membranous laryngitis," in which the mucous membrane of the larynx becomes inflamed, attended by the deposit of exudational matter in the form of a yellowish-white membrane upon its surface, there is none to which the human race is exposed more highly perilous to life or more baffling to the physician's resources in its management. The unspeakable ravages of this monstrous disease among the children of our land are well known alike to the medical profession and the laity. Though I shall not trouble the reader with a full description of its symptomatology, nevertheless, in view of the fact that the main object in its treatment is thereby rendered intelligible, to allude to the mode in which the disease accomplishes its deadly work seems to me to be pressing. The gravity of a particular case bears a pretty constant relation to the extent of membranous deposit, though to a smaller extent also to its seat. Thus when, as rarely happens, the exudation is confined to a portion of the larynx, the interference with the ingress and egress of the air during respiration is small, and the prognosis in such cases is not generally unfavorable; but if this deposit, as frequently occurs, should extend over the whole of the trachea, even reaching beyond the bifurcation of the bronchia, then on the other hand respiration, owing to the marked diminution of the calibre of the pipes, is greatly impeded, and as the result of successive attacks of dyspnœa of increasing violence, death ensues. This sad termination is produced in a way purely mechanical. To remove this offending pseudo-membrane by expectoration, either entire or by first causing its disintegration, is the physician's chief aim in grappling with true croup. The treatment of this affection is, however, divided into general and local, the latter constituting an essential part. Among the local means from time to time recommended by medical writers, the method of inhaling vapors which have been charged with different medicinal substances from an atomizer has been found to stand supreme, and the one substance which above all others has been received and transmitted by the medical profession with greatest favor is doubtless the vapor of limewater. Unquestionably an increase of moisture over the ordinary standard of relative humidity habitually present in the atmosphere of dwellings would be of eminent utility in the management of this affection. Hence it follows that plants under judicious regulations must be considered as applicable here, in the hope that they would not merely add to the general comfort of the patient, but beyond this prove to be more or less effective in macerating the false membrane and in mitigating the early inflammatory symptoms, in this manner, perhaps, indirectly serving to limit the deposition of the false exudation. At all events, as an element in the hygienic management of this disease, in which moisture in the air is so highly desirable, this use of plants, in the mind of the progressive medical man, will soon come to occupy a large place.

Wherever frequent and sudden vicissitudes of climate, with reference more particularly to the extent of saturation and the temperature-range, exist, the prevalence of laryngeal and bronchial affections may safely be inferred. The more commonly occurring among these diseases are known to medical writers by the terms acute and chronic laryngitis and bronchitis, the two former implying an inflammation of the whole or part of the mucous membrane of the larynx or voice-box, the two latter being of similar nature, having their seat in the bronchial tubes. There are certain other though comparatively rare varieties of the above-named forms of inflammation of these passages, to which brief allusion will hereafter be made, and a description of which would be out of place here; beside, we are solely concerned at present writing in making suggestions as to the question of the relation of living plants to the treatment of the above kinds of ailments. To commence, it is well to take a bird's-eye view of the treatment of catarrhal inflammation of the bronchial and laryngeal mucous membranes. Their handling is also usually divided into general and topical. In the milder shapes of acute laryngitis or bronchitis, however, appropriate general remedies together with ordinary sanitary precautions are all that is required. But the presence of a fair proportion of house-plants in the living- and sleeping-apartments of the patient suffering from such complaints would form an additional hygienic advantage of value, if to no other purpose than to obviate the unfavorable effects of dry furnace heat. Among the numerous instances of bronchitis, there are occasionally encountered by the physician those in which, on account of excessive irritability, cough becomes exceedingly troublesome, with scanty expectoration. Now, although such a state of affairs is in some degree presented by all cases of bronchitis during the early stages, we refer more especially to those last described, occupying extreme ground. In these instances a profusion of plants and flowers should be admitted both to the room occupied by the patient during the day and at night. Under these circumstances, the combined action of the plant-vapors and the ozone developed by the plants would, owing to their probable sedative effect and undoubted antiphlogistic action, tend materially to lessen morbid irritability and gradually reduce the catarrhal inflammation. Though this result is attained in a manner similar to that by the use of one of the many hand-atomizers, which are the product of the ingenuity of the human mind and much employed among physicians, unlike the latter, plant-exhalations possess the superior advantage of continuous operation, while, added to this, they not only serve to allay the accompanying functional disorders but also tend to give tonicity to the atmosphere of the home. It is, however, chiefly on account of their topical effects that they can be said to be capable of exercising a notably beneficial influence in this affection. To uphold the benefits to be derived from members of the floral household as in any sense constituting the exclusive dependence is far from the desire of the present writing, which is simply to represent them as valuable adjuvants.

But even more cogent than in the acute species are the reasons for suggesting a prudently selected collection of house-plants in the chronic or protracted forms of the disease. While less frequent in its occurrence than acute, chronic bronchitis is, nevertheless, not an uncommon complaint. Writers upon this disease usually describe three principal forms, each consisting of a considerable group of cases, while their several histories exhibit important variations with regard to the severity as well as the peculiar character of the symptoms. To describe lengthily the distinctive varieties of this affection is foreign to my object, and would be out of place in a work of this character, but to sketch briefly the chief characteristic features of each will answer a good purpose.

In the first place, let us consider ordinary chronic bronchitis, which at its commencement manifests itself in a mild form in winter only; but after several winters of recurring so-called "winter cough," the malady becomes permanently seated,—and now more or less cough is present throughout the seasons, with a predominance during the cold period. Of all forms, in this group the symptoms presented are the most variable, from slight cough and scanty expectoration, with little or no functional disturbance, on the one hand, to the most distressing paroxysms and free expectoration of yellowish-white or yellowish-green sputa, with considerable general disturbance, on the other.

The second class demanding notice is in every sense

typical. The chief abnormality of the membrane in this group is clearly expressed by the phrase, "dry bronchial irritation." The mucous membrane being exceedingly irritable, cough is frequent and severe, occurring chiefly in violent paroxysms, and is attended with the occasional expectoration of a small mass of viscid, pearl-colored mucus. In such, the breathing is constantly difficult, owing to the fact that the smaller tubes catch the brunt of the disease. In this form, bronchial catarrh is a most distressing malady, but, since taking its origin most frequently in the debilitating consequences of the patient's own previous intemperance, is to be classed with the long list of preventable diseases, on the one side, while less sympathy is, perhaps, called forth for this class of sufferers on the other. The third or last class to which attention is invited is termed bronchorrhœa, and, though occurring at different periods of life, it most frequently bechances those who have arrived at advanced life, being frequently found to be associated with disease of the heart. This form of bronchitis has for its cardinal distinguishing feature the expectoration of an abundant secretion, which may be either thick and glutinous or thin, fœtid, and transparent. Though usually very severe, the amount of cough present is sometimes very slight. To the patient, however, the one thing most detestable is the profuse expectoration.

Chronic bronchitis, of whatever form, is far less amenable to treatment than acute. After running the gauntlet of remedies both for internal administration and for inhalation, and finding no improvement, the physician frequently experiences no slight feeling of discouragement. Indeed, in a large proportion of these cases all efforts at effecting a cure are wasted on a forlorn hope; and hence, as there is no prospect of consummating a cure, the attendant must content himself with devices intended to place the patient in a condition of comfort, if this be possible. As every medical writer knows, of the sanitary conditions to be invoked in order to be eminently successful in the treatment of this exceedingly troublesome disease, there is none of higher importance than good pure air, with the proper degree of atmospheric humidity. To say that a right use of house-plants would meet these demands, can now scarcely excite dissent. In further consideration of the treatment of chronic inflammation of the mucous membrane of the bronchi, it is to be noted that amidst the multiplicity of remedial agents advised as having claim to special virtue in this condition, the preponderating number have been added to the list of substances for inhalation. Perhaps, next to a complete change of climate, these have proved their utility to be greater than the action of internal remedies.

Facts such as these, coincident with the circumstance that plant-exhalations—ozone and plant vapors—work out their effects in a manner which may justly be likened to that of the above class of remedies, though in silent energy having the marked advantage of being more continuous, it seems to me there is not a single theoretical reason to be enlisted against the use of flowering plants in every variety of this affection. The long-continued inhalation of an atmosphere such as described would, through its tranquillizing action upon the mucous membrane, produce results in some degree restorative.

If now, in addition to the faithful compliance with the recommendations concerning this measure, be also enjoined a fair amount of exercise in the open air whenever the weather permits, coupled with some attention to the matter of preserving proper habits of life, the reasonable expectation of the medical attendant or his unfortunate patient would perhaps be more than fulfilled. Of course, should the affection be intimately connected with other diseased conditions, these should receive due attention.

In conditions answering to the two last types of bronchitis above depicted, which types, the reader will remember, are termed "dry bronchial irritation" and bronchorrhœa, as well as in the severest forms of simple chronic bronchitis, medication seems to be of least benefit, and yet for certain good reasons these seem to be peculiarly adapted to the plant method of treatment. Thus it is in these categories of cases that the best authorities command the use of the different inhalations, or, their best devices having proved unproductive of good results, a change of climate is recommended, with pleasing issues in a certain number of instances. For such invalids the climate regarded as in the highest degree beneficial is one combining considerable humidity and a moderately high temperature, with slight fluctuations of both the elements named. Corresponding most nearly to this description, the climate of different regions of our own country, notably Southern California, Aiken in South Carolina, Thomasville in Southern Georgia, and the interior of Florida, are to be particularly mentioned.

From all that has been previously adduced respecting

the power of plant-transpiration to raise the degree of atmospheric saturation, the intelligent physician could, by giving some attention to the matter of accommodating the amount of vegetable life to the size of the living-room of a patient suffering from this disease, secure the extent of saturation most desirable in his climatic management. The temperature during the winter months, which is always the most trying season for this class of patients, is within-doors easily regulated by attention to heating and ventilation. Thus it is in our power to create, right in the home circle, the main climatic conditions most suitable for those ill with this harassing malady. Moreover, our home sanitarium may be said to possess certain advantages over the different reputed resorts to which the infirm are constantly ordered, which advantages will be pointed out hereafter. It, however, remains to be said in this connection that in the varied forms of chronic bronchitis it is perhaps more important than in any other class of conditions throughout the whole range of applicability of plants to disease, to maintain a uniform scale of relative humidity, or just such as can be furnished by a wise and careful selection of house-plants.

In cases of moderate severity of chronic bronchitis, the proportion of vegetable life laid down in the above formula for hygienic objects in health should be doubled, while in the second class, or cases of "dry bronchial irritation," for whose climatic treatment an atmosphere having decidedly sedative qualities is demanded, the former ratio should be trebled. Where irritability of the membrane is excessive, the use of inhalations of aqueous solutions more or less saturated with balsamic substances has numerous able advocates. By keeping alive, which can be done for a period of two weeks, branches from the species *Abies Canadensis*, or Norway spruce, in the patient's room in these instances, in connection with growing plants, thus impregnating the air constantly breathed by him, the terebinthinate vapors would have the best possible opportunity to exercise their well-known effects in substituting healthy for diseased processes, while the patient would no doubt experience less of troublesome cough and general discomfort as well. In order to procure the full benefits of the present mode of treatment of bronchial affections, the intimacy between the patient and his floral companions should be both unbroken and permanent, if possible. During the warm season, the same friendly connection can be kept up, if the patient be willing to take up their culture and to live among them, in the open air. To the poor, who are not exempt from this class of disorders, a method of relief such as here advocated cannot fail to be coveted as a blessing. The rooms occupied by the patient, in which the plants are kept, should be of good size, preferably, with a southern exposure. A neighboring greenhouse, to which he could have free access, might form a good substitute if conveniently located.

On reflecting that, as every medical man well knows, the sudden and notable changes in temperature and humidity, or, in other words, a severe and variable climate, constitutes the leading factor in the causal relation of the disease, surely an atmosphere changed by the liberal cultivation of house-plants, being mild, soothing, and above all, equable as to moisture and temperature, would speedily show no slight virtues as a means of obviating this dread affection.

In an article on chronic bronchitis ("System of Practical Medicine," edited by Dr. Wm. Pepper, vol. iii. p. 183), Dr. N. S. Davis has with much astuteness described still another category of subjects in the following curt but graphic terms. After asseverating that they are most frequently met with in persons of both sexes between twelve and twenty years of age, he continues: "They present a narrow, imperfectly developed chest, with so sensitive a condition of the bronchial mucous membrane that any trifling exposure to cold and damp air renews the vascular hyperæmia and cough until both become permanent, and the morbid process extends into the connective tissue of the pulmonary lobules, establishing what some call interstitial pneumonia, and others fibroid phthisis." With regard to the treatment of this condition, it is to be distinctly understood that it is not my design to attempt to underrate the importance of other measures, some of which have received the sanction of high authority, more particularly the inhalation of compressed air as practised by Dr. J. Solis Cohen, of Philadelphia, and warmly lauded by the late Dr. F. H. Davis, of Chicago, but to invite careful attention to the great promise held out by house-plants in such conditions. If this class of patients, it is to be noted, could have successfully thrown around them a certain safeguard against the liability to catch repeated "colds," they would soon find existence to be vastly more comfortable, and those later ill-fated developments above mentioned, and which latter place the life of the individual in jeopardy, could in great part be averted. Recalling the mild and equable properties of our house-plant clime, such a refuge as above depicted for sufferers from bronchitis in the living-chamber, can be confidently suggested as an abode for this not unimportant class of invalids, or still better, if agreeable to their tastes, let these subjects take up the occupation of florists, in which event they will be more constantly exposed to those gracious influences so devoutly to be wished for to promote their safety. It is quite probable that among the several plans of treatment heretofore devised for their management, none would give a greater return for the same moneyed consideration in the way of protection from future perils than the present.

Although there is as yet little evidence to confirm the rather novel measure in the treatment of chronic bronchial affections here proposed, namely, house-plants, it is to be especially observed that the inferences relating to its sanitary effects in this rather common and troublesome malady have been based upon the foundation of carefully demonstrated truths.

Finally, they have been commended in the sincere hope and belief that if put to the practical test of clinical experience in the before-named conditions, the result will be to establish the modest claims here advanced in their behalf completely.*

---

* Though having recently employed house-plants in a few instances of chronic bronchitis with satisfactory results, the histories of these cases are withheld for the reason that the patients are still under observation.

CHAPTER VII.

Living plants useful in consumption of the lungs—The latter disease very fatal, though not universally so—General facts relating to its etiology—Experiments tending to show its communicability from person to person—Professor R. Koch's discovery of the bacillus tuberculosis, which is the specific organism causing phthisis—His researches show that phthisis is infectious—Conditions under which the bacillus develops are peculiar—Treatment of phthisis discussed—No antidote to the bacillus found as yet—House-plants especially valuable in preventing the destructive work of this organism—Supporting evidence of a practical kind—The author's observations among florists—Cases confirmatory recorded by other writers—Requisites of health resorts for consumptives—Advantages of a home sanitarium—The relative amount of plant-growth required—The value of growing plants in confirmed phthisis—Cases illustrating the utility of plants in confirmed phthisis.

As health-giving agents, both on theoretical and clinical premises, growing plants offer the best assurance of success in that fell destroyer, consumption of the lungs. The supreme importance of this point demands that it shall secure careful attention. To enter upon a full consideration of the clinical history or the anatomical characters of this disease would be out of place here, and while on the one side these topics shall receive only incidental attention, as when of prime necessity to render intelligible the indications for treatment, on the other a fuller discussion of the various elements entering into the question of causation as well as the hygienic and climatic treatment seems pressing, if the reader is to be enabled to correctly estimate the value of house-plants as preventives and palliatives during the progress of an affection, the mere mention of whose name conveys to the popular mind an ominous purport. Indeed, from the most primitive times of which history gives us record, there has been current a deeply-implanted belief to the effect that invariably confirmed pulmonary consumption is hopelessly mortal. In this opinion the medical profession, to a man, shared also down to the time of Lænnec, a noted observer, who was the first to publish from his own pen some clinical evidence to show that cases having progressed to a stage in which excavations in the lungs occur, do sometimes take a favorable change and undergo a practical cure. Since that period, there have been numerous instances tending to establish clearly the fact that a limited number of cases, beyond a certain though variable stage, are no longer progressive, the patient continuing to live and to enjoy a tolerably comfortable existence, or even attaining old age, while a yet smaller percentage, as has been before intimated, either spontaneously or as the result of a recourse to approved sanitary and therapeutic measures, sustain a practical cure. It is undeniably to be classed as one of the most deadly diseases that the human race encounters, and is doubtless the greatest opprobrium to the medical profession. It is also a fact that admits of no gainsaying that of all the fatal ills it is the one causing more deaths than any other throughout the length and breadth of our land, being responsible for about fourteen per centum of deaths from all known causes. The manifold agencies which formerly were held to be most potent factors to produce this affection, have at the present day come to be very generally viewed as being but subsidiary.

Excepting the most recent writers upon the subject, all authors have been in the habit of enumerating a plexus of non-causes whose very complexity and numerical length evidenced the fact that the subject was shrouded in more or less mystery, and that the true or specific causative agency of the disease remained unrecognized. Relating to its etiology, certain general facts were, however, long ago fully substantiated. Thus the disease is most usual between the ages of twenty and thirty years, though it at least rarely occurs in advanced life. In temperate climes, whose changes of temperature are severe and sudden, it is more prevalent than in either the tropics or the cold meridians. The united testimony of numerous observers has also gone to show clearly that certain desiderata, such as habits, inherited predisposition, occupation, diet, constitutional condition, exercise, have more or less influence upon the appearance of the disease. The idea that this disease is communicable from one to another by contagion through the air to which a consumptive is exposed, already among the more ancient authors found quite able supporters. Within the two last decades the question has been exciting a rather lively controversy, resulting in the establishment of considerable evidence in favor of its being thus communicative. The first published experiments upon this subject were those conducted by Villemin, who in 1865 made the remarkable statement that by inserting tubercular matter taken from a patient under the skin of a healthy rabbit, he could successfully produce the total pathological lesions of the maturely-developed disease in the human subject. Perhaps the most decisive and at the same time interesting direct experiments in support of the infectious theory of phthisis, are those of Tappeimer, of Meran, in the Tyrol (*Lancet*, November 23, 1878, quoted by Hartshorne, Reynolds's System of Medicine, vol. ii. p. 116). He caused dogs to breathe for several hours daily the air of a chamber which had been impregnated by means of an atomizer with a mixture of phthisical sputa with water. After a period varying from twenty-five to forty-five days, all but one of eleven animals so treated were found, upon being killed, to have miliary tuberculosis of both lungs, most of them having some deposit also in the kidneys, and some in the liver and spleen. Microscopical examination accorded with the naked-eye appearances. The hypothesis of the specificity of the affection received further scientific confirmation from the ingenious investigations of a number of mycologists, who have been harmoniously successful in conveying the disease to healthy animals by mixing tuberculous matters with their food.

Now, from the array of reliable proof founded upon direct experiment, the indisputable cause of consumption of the lungs would seem to be a "specific virus," which proof does not, however, receive any satisfactory new light upon the important practical question, the isolation of the specific germ. It remained for the untiring energy of Professor Koch, of Berlin, to settle definitely the exact nature of the disease, and who by dint of patient industry in the execution of most ingenious and not less delicate culture-experiments, was enabled to indicate the specific organism, which he termed bacillus tuberculosis, causing tubercular consumption. In March, 1882, he published to the medical world an account of his skilful experiments, and although for a time after the announcement of his discovery its accuracy was from some quarters vehemently disputed, there can be no doubt whatever but that at this time it numbers among its advocates nearly every medical authority of eminent distinction, those so recently opposing the correctness of the theory themselves now forming recruits to reinforce the ranks of those already advocating its reliability.

A recent writer of wide fame, the late Professor Austin Flint ("System of Practical Medicine" (loc. cit.), vol. xix. p. 399), has the following statement: "Thus far the observations of competent medical mycologists are confirmatory of the results of the researches by Koch. It seems to be established that the so-called bacillus tuberculosis is uniformly present in tuberculous products, and as uniformly absent in other morbid products; that it is generally present in the sputa of phthisical patients, and never present in the sputa of non-phthisical patients, and that tubercular disease in animals may be produced by inoculation with organisms after cultivation has been sufficiently continued to eliminate all else pertaining to the tubercular product. On these data are based the conclusions that phthisis is an infectious disease."

While the results of the agreeable researches by Professor R. Koch furnish positive evidence that consumption of the lungs is an infectious disease, one thing is seen from the facts brought to light by the distinctive features of all clinical records of cases having their origin in contagion, to wit: that the disease is but feebly transmissible, or, in other words, for a person to contract it from a consumptive invalid close association for a long period of time continuously is essential. That the disease is very meagrely contagious is also shown by the fact that in point of frequency the disease is unparalleled by any other of a fatal character, and yet but an inconsiderable percentage of cases can be said to be the result of evident contagion. Clinical observations point to the fact that the greatest danger from infection lies in the exhaled breath, and from this is to be drawn the lesson that sleeping regularly with a consumptive is perilous.

These micro-organisms, it is to be remarked, living in the system under appropriate conditions become active, undergoing development and multiplication, which processes in time produce inflammatory action and consequent destructive changes in the lung-tissue. This latter fact, coupled with the one previously adduced showing the disease to be but feebly contagious, leaves no room for doubting but that the conditions under which it develops are very peculiar. What had been prior to the epoch occasioned by Koch's discovery regarded as causative agencies, have been since then looked upon as influences operating to prepare suitable conditions for the reception and injurious activity of this microbic intruder. The phenomenon here observed is at least suggestive of, if it be not identical with, the common custom exercised by the practical agriculturist, who makes ready the soil in accordance with the special crop he desires to cultivate, if he wishes to be reasonably certain of success. Further, as every one knows, under the presence of unfavorable climatic conditions or peculiarities of soil, certain species of plant life will not flourish.

Unfortunately for humanity, the bacillus tuberculosis is no such dismantled enemy; on the contrary, its ravages are so general that its presence in the human respirable medium must be wellnigh universal.

The vitally important practical question, how to combat successfully the deplorable work of this specific organism within the human system, challenges the serious attention of every practising physician. Since the recent disclosure of this parasitic intruder by Koch, the views relative to the treatment of phthisis have undergone considerable veering, and not a few competent investigators are already engaged in the work of discovering an antidote to this human foè, though up to the present moment the success attending their praiseworthy efforts does not furnish a basis for making a confident prediction. It is devoutly to be wished that the medical profession may not fall into the erroneous way of thinking that there can be no advantage in grappling with the disease until this much-hoped-for antidote shall have been found, and thus some of the most thoughtful measures and cardinal principles which have been the result of the accumulated experiences of the best medical minds, and which from time immemorial have guided the profession, be too much neglected.

In dealing with this disease, two main objects should engage the efforts of the clinician. The one aim already hinted at should be to attack the specific microbe itself, destroying or rendering it innocuous; the other should be to restrain those influences which promote the conditions of the air-passages favoring the propagation of the micro-organism producing the disease. Thus far, as has been shown, all efforts at finding an antidote to this organic germ within the human system have been practically "wasted on a forlorn hope," and from all the experimental evidence previously brought forward respecting the beneficial influences of house-plants upon the sanitary conditions of the atmosphere of our dwellings on the one hand, and their utility in the sick-chamber on the other, there are not sufficient facts to warrant the proposition that plant-exhalations are capable of annihilating the bacillus within the human body. More highly significant in this connection than the ozone evolved by the beautiful flowers are the moist vapors given off by the foliar organs of living plants, which vapors, by virtue of their constancy of action during respiration, keep up a healthy state of tonicity of the mucous surface of the respiratory tract, rendering these organs less liable to the influences which produce so-called "colds" in the common vernacular, or, in other words, overcoming the local conditions strongly favoring the commencement of the work of destruction by the bacillus tuberculosis. That this specific germ begins operations somewhere in the mucous membrane of the breathing tract there is no doubt whatever. And if, as before shown, living plants under proper treatment tend to maintain the bronchial mucous membrane throughout its whole extent in a healthy state, then the bacillus in the presence of plants must remain harmless, and the influence of the latter to perform signal service may be accepted with a feeling of confidence.

The words long ago uttered by John Locke, viz.,

"Prevention is better than cure, and far cheaper," certainly still hold with reference to pulmonary consumption. That half at least of all cases of phthisis are preventable is and long has been the harmonious opinion of medical writers of the foremost rank. The practical question how to prevent the development of consumption of the lungs becomes one of vital interest to every medical practitioner, in view of the foregoing facts relating to its fatality and unequal frequency. The family doctor very generally has the opportunity of knowing the inherited predisposition of his patrons, and it becomes his duty to point out the danger of this disease, and how to escape it, if he should be aware of the presence of such physical inheritance.

Hitherto we have put forward some of the theoretical considerations, the result of experimental work upon which the theory of the utility of growing plants in the prevention of phthisis is based. This hypothesis first received supporting evidence of an unequivocal character in my own published paper on "Hygienic and Therapeutic Relations of House-Plants" (*Philadelphia Medical Times*, May 8, 1880). About this period I opened a correspondence with a number of prominent clinicians, besides making inquiries of those with whom I chanced to come in contact, soliciting a brief statement of their observations with regard to the effect of growing plants upon the sick, with special reference to their influence in the monster disease under consideration. The almost unvarying responses proved to be in about the following terms: "I cannot help you, for my attention has never been directed to the points in question."

Finding that most of my correspondence yielded but barren results, I determined to avail myself of non-professional experience, and accordingly began visiting the gardens and florists of Philadelphia, requesting answers to a list of questions bearing upon the same point.

In this way brief histories of thirty florists, excepting in three subjects, whose histories were kindly furnished by Professor J. T. Rothrock, to whom my wants had been made known, were obtained. Twenty of these, with ages ranging from twenty-five to eighty years, were strong and vigorous, and had always enjoyed good health. Of the remaining number four were occasionally attacked with rheumatism of mild type, they themselves ascribing these invasions, and doubtless justly, to wettings, the result of carelessness while watering the plants, or from contact with the moistened leaves.

One of the gardeners, a lad aged fourteen years, had been engaged in a greenhouse for a year, working steadily ten hours daily. Prior to taking up this occupation he had been employed in a drug-store for a year. While thus at work his health failed notably, and he became pale and emaciated. It should be noted, however, that he had had poor health previously, though none of his organs could be said to be diseased. No sooner had he adopted the avocation of florist than a change in his condition set in, he began to improve in vigor, and I found him one year later to be the picture of robust health.

Another florist, aged thirty-one, says that prior to his going into the business he had "weak eyes," but as soon as he had followed the business of florist, eight years previous to my visits, his eyes began to improve, and in a few years entirely recovered.

Still another of the remaining ones had been subject to severe "colds" since he began to work among plants. But he admitted that he had been exceedingly indiscreet about clothing, etc., and in going from the hot-house into the open air.

Before speaking of the three remaining florists, whose records show the value of growing plants as agents to preserve human health, it will be noted that since making the above observations the histories of ten additional florists bearing upon this point have been carefully collected,—making a totality of forty cases.

One of the second series appeared elsewhere, and will be cited hereafter. Of the remainder, seven are to be classed with the twenty in the former series who were strong and vigorous and had always enjoyed excellent health. The two remaining of the second list died from consumption in advanced life, with strikingly similar clinical histories. Both subjects pursued the calling from early life, and continued in good health until, in consequence of the formation of habits of excessive dissipation, they were absent from their work the greater portion of the time. It was while in this state of marked intemperance and inattention to duty that this disease developed and rapidly proved fatal.

Unquestionably, such instances cannot in a spirit of fairness be reckoned as weighing either for or against the doctrine it is proposed to establish. At all events, they go equally far toward showing the danger of contracting the disease after becoming practically disassociated from living plants, as the inability of vegetation to prevent the disease in question.

The clinical notes of the single remaining florist of the last, as well as those of the first series not yet accounted for, were published more in detail in an article on "House-Plants and Lung-Disease" (*Transactions of Med. Soc. State of Penna.*, vol. xvi., 1883). Attention having previously been drawn to the subject of the excellent advantages of house-plants as preventives, cases strongly corroborating the same view were from various quarters reported, some of which latter were also chronicled in this paper, and will here again be recorded.

During the spring of 1882 there came under my professional care a patient, Mr. W., aged thirty-six years, giving the following interesting history: He had lost a father and two brothers from consumption. He stated that he had followed the occupation of florist and gardener from the age of fifteen years up to about one year previous to my having seen him; that he had worked almost continually among his plants from eight to ten hours daily, and that during this whole period had enjoyed fair health. He now abandoned his former calling, took a small store, and dealt only in cut flowers. After pursuing that business for a few months his general health gradually failed; cough set in, which gradually increased. Being of careless habits, the patient neglected this cough for a long time, and when he first applied to me the physical signs showed there was extensive softening of the upper lobe of the left lung and slight crepitation of the apex of the right one.

The future course of this case was typical of phthisis, terminating fatally about a year later. The father of the subject of the above sad sketch, although strongly predisposed by inherited constitutional tendencies, followed the occupation of florist from early life up to the age of sixty, and during all these years was in good health. When sixty years of age, while assisting at the erection of a church, he met with an accident which injured his ribs and disabled him for work. But a few months later he went into pulmonary consumption, which quickly proved fatal. Now, may not the fact that he was unable to be among his plants have had something to do with his last illness?

Another son died at the age of thirty-six years. He was engaged in gardening from boyhood up to within a year of his death, continually at work among his plants. During all of the time he followed this avocation he enjoyed fair health. A short time prior to his death he took a store in the same city, and almost simultaneously he became a victim to consumption, which caused his death in a short time. The fact that these two brothers had followed floriculture in good health for so many years, and so soon after making a change in their occupation they both fell into consumption of the lungs, is, to say the least, suggestive.

The father, who continued his calling as a florist until late in life, escaped the disease until as the result of an accident he was incapacitated for work, when he shared this sad fate with his unfortunate sons.

Is it not unreasonable to believe that had not these young men deserted their plants they might likewise have escaped the disease, at least so early in life?

A striking example of the value of house-plants in preventing the disease in question is recorded by Dr. Ely McClellan, U. S. A. (*Phila. Medical Times*, Feb. 26, 1881). He writes: "For the past three years there has been almost constantly under my observation a case which seems to corroborate the views expressed by Dr. J. M. Anders in his paper on the 'Hygienic and Therapeutic Relations of House-Plants.'

"E. M., a gentleman thirty years old, who belongs to a family in which there is a marked history of phthisis pulmonalis. His physical appearance would indicate that he might be subject to the disease, but he has as yet escaped its development. The history of the case involves the families of both the father and the mother. The father, although born of tubercular parents, escaped the disease, but the mother died at comparatively an early age, leaving a family of five children, four of whom have died of consumption. Of these children, three died between the ages of twenty and twenty-five years. One died in his thirty-ninth year, after a long illness, the last two years of which were under my observation. E. M. is the youngest of the family. His life, with the exception of the last eighteen months, has been devoted exclusively to sedentary pursuits. At twenty-three he married, and, as he was then engaged in an occupation which required his residence in an isolated locality, for both amusement and occupation his wife began the cultivation of house-plants. She soon became an enthusiast, and a profusion of plants, chiefly of the foliage varieties, accumulated in her house. As they resided in an exceedingly changeable climate, where during the cold months constant watchfulness was necessary for the preservation of plants, her bedroom and the adjoining sitting-room were arranged for that purpose.

"Before his marriage E. M., complained of, as he expressed it, a weakness of the chest and a constant liability to take cold. Since his marriage, with the exception of an occasional ailment, he has seemed a healthy man, and it is but reasonable to attribute his escape from the disease which had destroyed so many of his family to the fact that he lives and has lived for the past seven years in apartments well stocked with thrifty plants."

In an interesting communication on "Growing Plants in the Sick-Chamber" (*loc. cit.*), Dr. Hiram Corson, after referring to the case of a relative who during her long and happy life had derived marked advantage from her plants, which up to the time of her decease she continued to cultivate, he continues:

"Her cousin, a well-known botanist of Delaware County, Pennsylvania, whose only brother and sister died from consumption in middle age, lived among his plants to the age of seventy; and her brother, a well-known botanist of this country, who spent much time in his greenhouses, still lives at the age of ninety-four; while his daughter, who from early girlhood to the present time has been a botanist, and for more than forty years a practical cultivator of plants in hot- and green-houses, is strong and healthy as she now approaches her seventieth year."

From the extent and character of the practical, together with the experimental evidence above adduced, it will be granted doubtless that the dogma which claims for living plants a marked antiphlogistic action against the direst of all diseases, although not yet absolutely proved, rests upon no slender or insecure basis of proof.

Though the treatment of confirmed pulmonary consumption has in the past received the thoughtful attention of the best medical minds of any age, the subject has ever been and still is in the highest degree unsatisfactory. Unfortunately, no remedial measure, though many have been advised, has yet been found that can be depended upon as having any special influence upon the morbid lesional processes accompanying the various stages of the affection. Perhaps the best results we are in a position to hope for, are: to arrest in a small percentage of cases the onward march of the disease to a fatal issue, to palliate in the remainder or larger percentage of cases, symptoms, such as troublesome cough, diarrhœa, hemorrhage from the lungs, and so forth, and to build up the general system. But it is not my intention to underestimate the importance of medicinal measures, since to effect the objects mentioned is an office not to be despised. There are also certain hygienic measures —proper diet, out-of-door exercise, for example—whose significance should not be overlooked. According to the unanimous opinion of the foremost authorities, the best advantages to the interests of this class of invalids are usually derived from a judicious change of air. But to enter upon a full discussion of the treatment of pulmonary phthisis here is not my purpose; on the other part, however, since our home floral sanitarium previously described embraces many happy influences common to all leading health stations, certain broad considerations touching the latter become importunate. The idea is pretty generally received that in making a change of climate it is necessary to go to points long distances from home, than which, however, there could be none more gratuitous. It cannot be denied, too, that among the many which have been, and still are being, pressed upon the attention of the medical profession and a gullible public, few health resorts have enjoyed more than a brief popularity. In strict justice it is to be observed that many so-called health stations are in reality comparable only to the patent nostrums which certain unprincipled parties are continually foisting upon the drug market, they having little more to commend themselves than the latter; with them, too, they likewise soon sink into merited oblivion. There are other regions whose climatic effects upon well-selected cases of phthisis have proved their power for good to be most estimable. Owing to the conflicting results from the climes ordinarily met with; it would seem to be congruous at this point to inquire what constitutes the requisites of an appropriate climate for the consumptive sufferer. In brief, the elements dryness, equability, and purity are by unanimous consent of nearly all authorities regarded as the most essential desiderata. And the localities which produce the most favorable results with reference to the element, temperature, occupy the two extremes, being either hot or very cold, with the balance of testimony in favor of the latter. In cold climates at high altitudes, though the qualities purity and dryness obtain, equability does not; on the contrary, the daily temperature range, owing to active nocturnal terrestrial radiation, is very great; this circumstance forming the chief objection to high and dry climes. On the other hand, a natural equable climate is almost invariably found to accompany a high temperature. Florida, for example, has considerable humidity, which latter element also gives it a more or less relaxing influence. But the various meteorological elements of the diverse climates usually frequented by consumptive invalids will, when treating in a subsequent chapter of the "Sanitary Influences of Forests," be discussed more lengthily.

Referring again to our floral sanitarium, and recapitulating the most important desiderata upon which its claims as such are based, the reader will remember that the atmosphere of this resort possesses certain unmistakable advantages of remarkable excellence. If few noted health stations are equally so, none are, perhaps, more favored with the most desirable conditions of climate. In the first place, the element of equability, or uniformity of the degree of moisture in the air, as well as of temperature, may, as previously demonstrated, be here attained. Though this pleasant retreat cannot afford a cold climate, at the temperature of ordinary living-apartments (65° Fahr.), especially during the winter season, the effect would not be to enervate; in other words, something comparable to a mild, temperate, out-of-door climate would be thus secured. Again, the temperature within-doors could be readily kept at a higher standard, if desirable. During the hot months of midsummer the patient should spend a goodly portion of his hours in the society of his plants in the open air, or seek shady nooks or the balmy air of a neighboring forest, or, if practicable, the nearest mountain resort of low or medium altitude, where measurably good culinary and other home comforts are obtainable. In behalf of those who cannot bear the expense accompanying a brief sojourn to the nearest mountain resort, or at some more quiet rural retirement, for their comforting assurance the fact should be noted that the effect of a fair proportion of house-plants in a room in summer is to reduce, in consequence of the moist vapors given off, the temperature at least from 4° to 6° Fahr. Those in the latter class who cannot escape the oppressive midsummer heat of our cities, should take up the practice of floriculture both in-doors and out. A few hours daily spent in a greenhouse would prove highly beneficial to such, if conveniently located.

Thus far our miniature health resort for stay-at-homes has, it is seen, answered to all the indispensable requirements of the climate best adapted to consumptives, save one, namely, dryness. In the first place, the ablest and most earnest advocates of a dry and rarefied air acknowledge the existence of a large class of consumptive invalids not suited to such climatic conditions. This category comprises those in the later stages of the affection; those in whom the disease manifests a tendency to progress rapidly with the frequent occurrence of hæmoptysis, or all those suffering from marked debility, which condition operates to preclude the possibility of becoming acclimated. To such the sagacious physician would not recommend a Colorado climate in the hope of benefiting his patients; on the contrary, cases belonging to this category demand a more genial climate, with a fair degree of saturation. In considering the element of dryness, therefore, the above large percentage of cases, as well as the equally large class of those who, for financial or other reasons, cannot contemplate such a course, are practically excluded. The writer has no intention of denying the incalculable value of this meteorological component in carefully-chosen examples of chronic forms of phthisis, and especially in the earlier stages, since to do so would be to oppose the favorable results of numerous trials among patients who, at the advice of their physician, have in recent time made choice of the high and dry regions of Colorado and New Mexico. But the practice of indiscriminately sending phthisical patients to them is certainly to be deprecated. For the class of invalids demanding an arid climate, or one answering to the above description, and who are not circumstanced so as to make the needed change of air, the employment of growing plants in such ratio as will not produce a degree of humidity above the normal limit, or that previously recommended as most fully conducive to health, would prove serviceable. Medical men of experience are of one opinion respecting the observation that females do not, for physical reasons, tolerate well a cold climate; while few are so favorably situated as to command the opportunity to have recourse to a Colorado resort. To such also come the blessings of a home sanitarium. There is here a pleasing concurrence, in great part, owing to the circumstance that a greater portion of the lives of the female than that of the male sex is spent in-doors, and in some part to the fact that a love for flowers appears to be more strongly indigenous and their culture more congenial to the tastes of the former than the latter. The pursuit of health by cordially embracing a course according so gratefully with their refined tastes and moral purity, will further commend itself to the practically-minded reader on account of its inexpensiveness, being within reach of all. Plant humidity, it should be here noted, is not open to the grave objections which are known to hold against humidity of an out-of-door climate. Thus, at resorts whose atmospheres contain considerable humidity, but small fluctuations in the temperature are certain to produce a chilling effect, which is decidedly harmful to invalids in search of lost health. Again, at resorts answering to the above description, the temperature is usually so high as to have, in combination with the moisture present, a relaxing effect. As has already been intimated, the temperature of our home sanitarium can within certain defined limits be easily regulated, not only with reference to mean elevation, but also the highly-important matter of daily oscillations, in this manner averting chilling influences. Moreover, as elsewhere argued with good show of reason, the plant vapors may be assumed to be widely different from those evaporated from inorganic matter and from bodies of water, being purified and endowed with medical properties by passing through the plant. It is quite reasonable to suppose that with the rapid transpiration of aqueous vapor from a plant there are active principles peculiar to the species floating in its life-current, which also assume the gaseous form and are held in solution by the vapor given off, thus medicating it. The observation has been made that children playing among our common poppy-plants will manifest signs indicating the physiological effects of opium, which must have gained entrance to the system through the inhaled air. That the air of the pine and hemlock forests is impregnated with the vapor of turpentine is well known, and the value of which vapor for giving relief to the pulmonary invalid has long been established. Doubtless all the species belonging to the large order of conifera give off medicinal agents. Plants, therefore, are Nature's faithful and perfect atomizers, whose vapors are perhaps capable of an equally high and useful purpose, respecting their therapeutic application, with those that are the products of the ingenuity of man.

Perhaps some of the superior advantages of a home-sanitarium would become more prominently apparent if some of the evident and acknowledged disadvantages of ordinary health resorts were briefly enumerated. In order to derive benefit that shall be enduring, the patient must make his new abode more or less permanent, not less than two or more years; and this prolonged separation from home and former associations involves issues of great significance to his pecuniary interest and subsequent comfort, besides producing anxiety of mind, granted that his health would thereby be restored. The invalid in not a few instances, soon after reaching his new habitat which he had confidently expected would prove a source from whence he should derive new vigor and returning health, begins to suffer from home-sickness, and in consequence of this, before becoming acclimated, but after having received the unpleasant effects experienced on his advent, and the fatigue of a long journey, sets out for home, and after reaching that blissful spot, his physician usually finds his physical condition far from being as favorable as when he first left home. But though the patient should remain long enough to receive benefit, too often a trial of a reputed health station brings only disappointment, and the consumptive is rendered more miserable by the annoyance of travel and the anxiety of being separated from all the endearing relations of home.

The difficulty in nearly all, and utter impossibility in many cases, of obtaining home comforts at the various resorts in different climates, however genial, form an important topic for the consideration of the practising physician, but cannot at present writing receive the attention it so richly deserves. It should, however, be noted that the one condition which more than any other counter-influences the beneficial effects of the balmiest climate, is bad cookery. Finally, there is often a lack of opportunity for the patient to find satisfactory methods of enjoyment or congenial society.

On the other hand, to have always at hand and readily available so complete and withal so agreeable a health resort at home as that afforded by a living-apartment well supplied with growing plants and flowers, must prove to the despairing invalid an inestimable boon.

Wherever the weather during the cold season is inclement, the stay-at-home who resorts to our miniature shelter is at disadvantage with regard to a matter which is vitally significant, namely, exercise in the open air. As has been before intimated, the patient, when practicable, should adopt the work of a practical floriculturist, which would in itself insure some degree of exercise, though not to any great extent in winter, when the plants, as in our meridian at Philadelphia, must be cultivated solely within-doors. But if the room be of good size, as it should be, not less than twelve by twenty feet, including, if practicable, an adjoining room, and having two or more windows with a southern exposure, thus admitting an abundance of sunlight, and if, as has been above shown by physiological experiment, the meteorological conditions of the air of our plant-refuge strikingly resemble a genial, temperate out-of-door climate, then a jaunt through such apartments would not prove to be without virtue. A still better measure to the end of securing the much-needed exercise is afforded by the graceful arrangement, before referred to, displayed in the beautiful solarium of the New York Hospital. This would furnish excellent opportunity for a ramble among green foliage and flowering vegetation. In view of the premises established in behalf of vegetable life and its effects upon several classes of invalids, the suggestion that every large city or even small town should be furnished with a certain number, according to the population, of health-giving retreats of this character would not be untimely.

While the patient, on account of the inclemency of the weather, is prohibited from practising daily exercise in the open air, the above recommendations might be supplemented by resorting to such gentle methods of physical exercise in-doors as the use of a simple rubber band with handles, which, besides exercising the muscles of the upper portion of the body, expands the chest; or, still better, a rubber ball such as used at "wall-ball;" during which playful exercise nearly every group of muscles of the system is brought into activity.

Of course, when the state of the weather and the strength of the patient will admit of it, he should take daily brisk walks and other forms of exercise out of doors. During the warm season the best effects from the growing plants are to be obtained by their additional culture, and spending as much time as possible among them, in the open air. In this connection there is no other question of greater significance demanding attention than that pertaining to the judicious selection of varieties, so as to insure success in their cultivation and yet to obtain their full benefit as hygienic agencies, and for the information upon this branch of the subject the reader is referred to a subsequent chapter, which discusses all essential points pertaining to practical floriculture.

Not less vitally important is the question of the proper proportion of plant life in these instances. As a broad rule, it may be said a greater profusion of plants—blooming and non-blooming—is essential in the advanced stages of the disease, as when cavities exist in the lungs or there is present marked hectic fever or a highly-sensitive nervous system, than in the earlier stages of chronic phthisis, as well as when cultivated for their effects as preventive agents. For the latter classes the ratio laid down in the previous chapter for sanitary objects in health should at least be doubled, while in the former classes or those in the last stages of the disease, who require a warm, genial atmosphere with considerable humidity, this amount in relation to the cubic space of the room or rooms should again be doubled, giving us four times the amount recommended as the best standard for living- and sleeping-rooms.

Owing to particular exigencies of individual cases, the proper relation of plant growth can be only approximately stated; in short, this question should always be determined by the judgment of the attending physician or some practical scientific interpreter.

Having antecedently set forth by *a priori* reasoning the probable utility of growing plants in the treatment of lung-disease from the side of natural history as well as experimental exploration, the author wishes to append some illustrative examples, which are taken from the records of cases occurring in the experience of certain standard medical writers and in his own (*loc. cit.*), showing indisputably the signal value of house-plants as remedial agents in conditions of chronic phthisis.

Case I.—The history of an interesting occurrence of chronic phthisis, of which I shall here give the more pronounced details, was received from my friend Dr. Hiram Corson, of Conshohocken, Pennsylvania. He writes: " My mother, her two sisters, and only brother, all died of consumption under fifty years of age. All the children of my mother's brother, though they lived to a good age and enjoyed good health, finally died of consumption. On my father's side there was not a taint of any disease, but great strength and vigor.

Three of my brothers—active, energetic men until within a few years of their death—died of consumption at the ages of fifty-five, fifty-seven, and seventy-eight, respectively, and a sister died of the same disease at sixty-six. I mention those cases to show that the germs of the disease were with the family.

"Thirty years ago, my eldest sister, then about fifty years of age, was reported by her physician, Dr. J. P., a victim of tubercular consumption, to which she would succumb before the coming summer. She was a lover of plants and flowers, and cultivated them in-doors and out. The spring saw her again working among her plants, and the winter found her confined to the house. Visitors and friends often spoke to her of the impropriety of having so many growing plants in her room, reminding her of the tradition that they were injurious. Still, every spring found her again on her feet in the yard and garden, nursing her plants, and every winter confined to her room. And thus she lived, year after year, until two years ago, when at the age of eighty-five she passed away. I have seen a few others have plants growing and blooming in their chambers, but never one who so lived among them as did my sister. Winter after winter we looked for her death, the cough, expectoration, and weakness justifying our apprehensions, and yet her eighty-fifth year found her cheerful and happy, living among her plants and enjoying the society of her friends. May we not believe that the vast exhalation from these plants, water purified and medicated by their vital chemistry, prolonged her life?"

Case II.—Mr. W., æt. thirty-five, has been in business as a florist for twenty years, and is among his plants ten hours daily. Phthisis is hereditary in his father's family, and my informant himself (Mr. W.) has long since been pronounced to be consumpted by his physician, Dr. S. R.* He states, however, that he has always enjoyed fair health, except simply the annoyance of slight cough and a little expectoration. He is still nursing his plants and enjoying life.

Case III.—There appeared in the *Christian Advocate* for July 29, 1880, by its medical editor, Dr. Pilcher, the following history, which, if not fully confirmatory, is at least suggestive of the foregoing favorable results.

"Two years since there was under my care one whose prolonged cough and repeated attacks of bleeding from the lungs gave every promise of speedy death from consumption. As he rallied from the last attack of bleeding and was able to crawl about again, in order that he might have the benefit of the tonic action of the sunlight he was advised to pass several days daily basking in the sun in the hot-house of a neighboring florist. This he faithfully did during the spring until the weather made it possible to spend his time in the park. In addition to this, all the usual measures which are accepted as of value in such condition were adopted, but the sun-baths (in the greenhouse) were especially insisted upon as of prime importance. The sick man steadily improved. His cough became less troublesome. His strength returned. No further bleeding occurred. At the end of several months he resumed work at his place, and

---

* The correctness of this diagnosis (fibroid phthisis) was corroborated by a personal physical examination by the writer.

now for over a year has been apparently well, pursuing a trying avocation without interruption." It should be stated that the above clinical record of Dr. Pilcher's case was published as tending to confirm the author's views relative to the sanitary value of growing plants in affections of the lungs.

Case IV. occurred recently in the writer's own practice. The patient, Miss S., aged twenty years, was the eldest of three daughters in a very comfortable family. There was a marked history of phthisis and scrofulosus in the family antecedents of both the father and the mother; parents, however, living and enjoying fair health. At the age of ten our patient had necrosis of the femur as the result of a sprain, lasting a year, during which time a few spiculæ of bone were thrown off spontaneously. Subsequently the leg kindly healed and gave her no further trouble. She had been a sufferer for several years from atonic dyspepsia, associated with habitual constipation. During the winter prior to her illness she had been subject to frequent colds on the chest, which, however, made no impression upon her general health. May 1 she contracted an ordinary " cold," and treated it apparently successfully with domestic remedies. About a month later she again caught a severe "cold," but now domestic medication proved to be of no avail, and, after a trial of one month, the cough meanwhile becoming more and more troublesome, I was consulted. At this period, July 14, she complained greatly of a tickling sensation in the region of the larynx, which sensation, according to her statement, was present from the beginning, and gave rise to hacking cough. There was scanty expectoration of mucus, the appetite was poor, and digestion greatly impaired. The physical signs were almost negative, consisting of slight dulness on percussion over the left apex, and feeble respiratory murmur and occasionally crepitation was heard during inspiration by auscultation over the same area. A change of residence was strongly advised, and she was accordingly sent to the Blue Ridge to live with the family of a friend, under the care of a reputable physician. Here she remained seven weeks. On her return in the autumn her condition was found to be worse in every respect. Anæmia was pronounced, and weakness equally so, with slight loss in bodily weight. The physical signs were vastly more marked. Despite the employment of suitable internal remedial measures and careful attention to diet, the pathological changes in the lungs steadily grew more pronounced, evidences of the process of excavation already appearing. November 1 the digestive organs rather abruptly became greatly deranged, with still further reduction in her general strength. This excited grave apprehensions lest the approaching winter season should to a great degree aggravate her disease and compel her to be constantly confined to her private apartments, with the usual consequences of such practice. A change to some warmer climate was contemplated, but it was finally decided between Dr. L. Starr, my consultant, and myself that her strength was too feeble to admit of a journey to a southern climate. Her condition was unpromising: pulse varying from 110 to 120 beats per minute; hectic fever quite marked; great weakness, and emaciation progressive. She was now able to walk only two or three squares with the most strenuous efforts. The symptoms referable to the larynx were very distressing, the patient complaining greatly of dryness and burning pain in that region, there being undoubted tubercular laryngitis. This was her unfortunate condition November 5, when it was decided to fill the living- and sleeping-rooms with thrifty foliage-plants. The second story front room was selected, its dimensions being twelve by fifteen feet, and three dozen plants, chiefly of the foliage varieties, were introduced, with an average leaf-surface of about four square feet. The apartments were heated by a hot-air furnace. The atmosphere of the room was at once decidedly changed and rendered strikingly agreeable by the plants, besides the room being much more cheerful and attractive. Thus she lived almost exclusively among her plants during the whole winter season. The temperature was kept at from 68° to 70° Fahr. The internal treatment during her confinement was that usually adopted in like cases. Spring, May 1, found her not any more reduced in flesh and strength than when she betook herself to her room in the fall. The weather having become fine, she was advised to take gentle exercise out of doors, on fine days a drive to Fairmount Park being a part of her daily recreation. Meanwhile the local lesions had to some extent advanced, and a cavity of some size had formed in the left lung, while the right also had become involved, as evidenced by crepitant râles heard over about one-fourth of its whole extent. The months of July and August were spent in the country. After returning home at the beginning of September, diarrhœa, which had troubled her somewhat during the hot term, continued despite the most active treatment until October 5, when death hastily carried off my friend and patient.

Now, as to the effect of the plants on our patient's condition. In the first place it must be borne in mind that before this method of treatment was adopted the disease already had assumed a pronounced form, having been pretty far advanced as regards the local lesions, and hence a cure was out of the question, and it was scarcely to be expected that the progress of the disease could be even arrested; but the object was to try to alleviate urgent symptoms, to prolong life, and make it as comfortable as possible. These expectations were fully realized. After entering the floral retreat, the patient at once experienced an agreeable sense of relief, existence becoming comfortable. It will have been observed that the general strength underwent no change during four months of absolute confinement. Perhaps no better evidence of the happy effects of the plant-exhalations upon the atmosphere of the room could be adduced than the fact that the patient was frequently heard to declare, when in any of the other rooms of the house for a few minutes only, that she felt vastly more uncomfortable than in her own apartment, and should be obliged to return to it.

But to arrive at a correct estimate of the usefulness of the plants in this patient, we shall have to pass in review their effects upon the various symptoms in detail. The almost constant laryngeal irritation of which the patient had complained so much was diminished in a marked degree. The cough was less frequent and caused less pain than before she repaired to this artificial bower, this marked relief being probably due to the favorable influence of the plant atmosphere upon the diseased laryngeal and bronchial mucous membranes. The hectic flush to which our patient was a victim, though nearly so well marked, was better borne while in the room with her floral comrades. There can be no doubt, however, that the greatest service rendered by the plants in this case was the good degree of grateful comfort they brought, apparently independently of their effects upon individual symptoms severally, due to their purifying and freshening influence upon the atmosphere.

Case V.—The writer's note-book furnishes the following brief history, which has not previously been published: M. H., aged thirty-three years, whose family antecedents gave no history of tubercular phthisis, applied to me in February, 1883. From boyhood to the date of this visit he had pursued carpet-weaving for a livelihood, and, though not actually robust, from a still earlier period of his life had, up to the date of the onset of his present illness, about a month previous to his first visit, possessed good health. His condition when he consulted me was the result of catching a heavy cold. His symptoms were troublesome cough, accompanied by slight expectoration of a yellowish-white color and tenacious character. There had been neither loss of flesh nor febrile disturbance, but the appetite had failed and the general health of the patient had begun to decline. A slight hemorrhage from the lungs, which occurred but two days previous, caused him to be much disturbed.

A physical exploration of the lungs revealed a small

area of fulness on percussion and the existence of slight crepitation over the same on auscultation. The evidences of commencing phthisis pulmonalis were thought to be complete.

Believing the patient's condition to be one in which growing plants would be serviceable, this plan of treatment was instituted after being assured by my patient that all its details would be faithfully complied with. Forthwith both living- and sleeping-chambers were suitably supplied with thrifty foliage and flowering plants, and now for a period of about four months his time was nearly wholly spent in company with his newly-welcomed guests. Since the patient's home afforded no rooms of a desirable size, however, and since there was located but a short distance from his abode a greenhouse to which access was, upon request, kindly granted, he was counselled to spend at least three hours daily luxuriating in the sunshine of the greenhouse, where the united action of plant-exhalations and sunlight had the most favorable opportunity of exercising a beneficent influence. Having continued his relations with the plants for one month, the cough began to lessen; likewise the expectoration. The bleeding from the lungs did not recur, and the general strength of the patient began to show improvement. At the end of the next two months the physical signs were upon examination found to be entirely absent, and coughing was the rarest event. In short, he was substantially sound. As employment was not then open to him he was ordered to go to the country for the heated term, which he did a month later, returning in September and looking quite hale. He resumed work, and maintained good health until last seen, about one year later.

In the present chapter there have been recorded a number of examples tending to show the value of plants as preventive and remedial agencies in phthisis; too few, perhaps, to furnish a reliable basis for definite conclusions, still they are of such unquestionable importance as to call for more extended observation in the same direction, with the purpose either of establishing or disproving the premises here contended for. That they can rise to the position of a specific in this dread disease is not claimed for living plants, but it would seem that they are capable of bringing about an arrest of the progress of the disease in some instances, or even, very rarely, a cure, with the aid of medicinal and sanitary measures advised by high authority for such conditions,—for in looking back at the cases reported the reader will observe that in two an apparent cure was effected by the combined action of the sun-baths and plant-exhalations. In two others the disease was to such a degree controlled as that life was prolonged and a comfortable existence maintained indefinitely. Lastly, from the unanimous testimony thus far collected, the ability of growing plants under proper adjustment to prevent its invasion is quite probable.

CHAPTER VIII.

Soil for potting flowers—It should be composed of decaying sods—It should be porous—Fertilizers—They should be well decayed—Plants requiring special soils—Chemical fertilizers—Heat and moisture—Continuous supply of moisture to the roots generally necessary—The proper temperature variable—Plants that love light and warmth and those loving shade—Air of living-rooms congenial to most plants—Roots love darkness—Feeding roots keep near the surface of the soil—Watering of plants—This supplies oxygen—Sulphurous gases injurious—Temperature of water—Potting—Necessity of holes for drainage—Cuttings—Training of plants—New varieties from seed—Insects and disease—The window garden—Flowers suited to in-door cultivation—Aquariums—The greenhouse and conservatory—Designs for the latter—Methods of heating—Out-door gardening—Rosery.

WHAT kind of soil shall I use? is the first question with one who would grow flowers. Gardeners of the past age were more particular than those of the present time. Their potting-sheds were the counterpart of an apothecary's store. Divisional boxes were prepared for no end of material, and for potting the various classes of plants the mixtures were as numerous and the parts as accurately weighed out as if prepared by an apothecary on the prescription of a physician. Modern gardeners have fallen into the opposite extreme, and it is not unusual to read that one kind of soil is good enough for everything. Certainly under this belief plant-growing has deteriorated. It is rare that we see the fine specimens of skilful culture that the gardeners of the past generation delighted in. After all, the exact proportions or mixtures, the best kind of soil to suit any one class of plants must come more from experience than from teaching. The true plant-lover soon learns to detect the preference of the plant, yet some attention must be paid to the character of the soil. Gardeners generally consider the essential body of the material should be composed of rotten sods. This is usually the upper portion or surface of a grassy meadow, and if it is from an old pasture that has been several years in grass it is all the better. This is taken off about three or four inches deep, according as it may be full of old roots or not,—for it is the mass of roots furnished by the grass that seems to give this kind of soil its good reputation. If very full of old roots, it may be taken off deeper than if not abundant. It is the greater quantity of roots that an old pasture furnishes that makes it the best soil for potting plants. If a piece of grassy ground or old sod is not too hard, the waste-heap of the gardener, on which the weeds from the summer's work have been thrown, will furnish very good potting material. Indeed, some good flower-growers prefer this. The chief object is to get for the main body of the soil earth that has an abundance of small roots decaying through it. When the sod can be had, it is generally piled in a heap for the greater part of one season, in order to start the roots on the road to decay. In many cases this would furnish all that would be required for a good potting soil, but generally it would be too heavy or stiff. Then it is lightened by the addition of sharp sand. Aside from this, some enriching manure is advantageous. Thus we often have this formula for good potting soil: one-third loam, one-third sand, and one-third well-decayed manure. From what has been said, it will be clear that what is needed is a soil that is somewhat open, and, if heavy, the sand is to lighten it. If poor, the manure is to enrich it. In some cases it will be rich enough and light enough with no additions. If any sand or manure be added, the proportions must vary with the judgment of the plant-grower. There is much difference of opinion among plant-growers as to the best kind of manure to put with earth to make good potting soil. The general conclusion is that cow manure is the best. It ought at least to be one year old, and in such a condition when used that it will reduce to powder. Horse manure would be regarded as the next in order, but they all must come under the term well decayed. Leaf mould is an excellent material for potting soil, but this should be at least three years old, unless it has been under circumstances favorable to a very rapid decay. In old times, before steam and hot water had been so generally employed in heating garden structures, hot-beds were formed of fermenting materials; leaves and other vegetable substances thus employed soon decayed, and then furnished the chief enriching material used by florists. Hot-bed manure is now rarely to be had. Leaf mould fresh from the woods is often employed, but generally fermentation has not quite done its work. In the florists' language, it is too poor, and it is best to let it remain a year or so before using it. It is this lack of complete fermentation that makes it so necessary that all manure used should be well decayed. After all, this is, in technical language, the great aim of the flower-grower, to have his soil "sweet." There should be no musty, mushroomy smell about it,—it should have a spongy, or, as the professional man would say, a "fibrous texture," and it should be "porous" by the help of sand or similar material, to enable water to pass rapidly through. With these general hints, the flower-lover will soon learn to prepare a first-class potting soil. Some plants are, however, fastidious, and special soils have to be prepared for them. Those which have an abundance of hair-like roots, such as azaleas, rhododendrons, and ericaceous or heath-like plants, generally require a particularly spongy soil, in which these roots may roam around in cool, air-filled cavities, and for these what the gardener calls peat is very desirable. This need not be exactly the peat of the Old World, often used for fuel, but the dark, decayed mass of moss, roots, and sand that is so common in "Jersey swamps" or pine barrens. This can be had of most dealers in florists' supplies by the barrel, and, though the experienced florist learns how to prepare the soil that shall be a good substitute for it, the younger amateur will find a small quantity a very useful aid in successful culture. A small quantity of coarse mats, and a box of broken brick or old flower-pots, will furnish a very good outfit in the potting-room for one who would grow flowers.

A small quantity of special fertilizing material may be kept on hand for use occasionally. The clearing of the hog-pen, when well decayed, has been found of great benefit to the growth of coarse, leafy plants, such as geraniums and pelargoniums, and those who have taken pride in growing superior specimens of those plants for exhibition purposes have found great help in its application. Poudrette or mixed soil, after it has been a year in the earth-covered heap, is a very superior fertilizer for pot flowers; but it is very powerful in its action, and a couple of ounces or so is quite enough for the earth that would fill a six-inch pot. Guano, or the sweepings of the dove-cote or chicken-yard, is also an extremely powerful fertilizer, and even less proportion in the case of night soil is all one would require. All these very active fertilizers are more frequently used for sprinkling on the surface—top-dressing, florists call it—of the soil, than for mixing generally through it. Bouvardias seem especially to luxuriate in top-dressings of highly-concentrated manures.

Chemical fertilizers, such as potash, soda, salt, ammonia, and similar articles, are often used to great advantage by skilful plant-growers, but the novice should employ them very cautiously at first, and observe the effect on the growth before using them to any great extent. They are very useful in the hands of experience. A great variety of plant-diseases come from fungous plants feeding on the roots, and these materials, judiciously used, often prove the best correctives.

Heat and moisture are so intimately connected that it is requisite to consider them together. Most treatises on gardening tell us that there is a continual evaporation of moisture from the leaves of plants, and that water must be applied to make good this waste. But evaporation is scarcely the term to apply, for the process of life is nearly akin in both plants and animals. Animals do not evaporate moisture, they perspire. Plants transpire,—but we might nearly as well apply the same term to both. The process of life is one of combustion, and perspiration in animals or transpiration in plants carries off the surplus heat. If there be not water to take the place of the moisture transpired, the plant will dry up, and this may occur from dry cold winds as well as from an excess of temperature. Plants, then, must have a continuous supply of moisture, as well as some degree of light and heat, in order to keep them in good health.

It is extremely difficult to give exact directions for practice, on account of nature having so arranged things that what may be called the normal conditions vary with each class. Some plants will live for months without water; others, almost aquatics, must have water continually; and while some must have a high temperature, others are in perfection where the temperature is but little above the freezing-point. Hence, books on flowers usually tell the reader to water plants only when they need it, and to be careful not to keep plants in too high, too low, too shady, or too sunny a place. One learns but little from this advice, for what is too much or too little is just what the novice wants to know. As a general rule, those plants that have hairy stems or leaves transpire freely, and love light. These may generally be selected for the warmest and sunniest places. It can scarcely be too light for heliotrope, coleus, geraniums, verbenas, or plants of that class. Begonias, and similar plants with smooth leaves, will do in partial shade; while large, thin-leaved, smooth plants, like the Arum family of plants, will do well in deep shade. Nature, however, seems to delight in paradoxes. Exceptions to these rules are not uncommon. The carnation is a smooth-leaved plant, and yet few plants love light more; and the cactus, fig-marigold, and succulents or fleshy-leaved plants generally, are of this character. But in arranging for these exceptions to rule, nature has placed but few channels for transpiration in their leaves.

At one time it was supposed that a moist atmosphere was an essential element in the successful growth of plants, and hence arose no end of schemes and labor for securing in plant-houses an atmosphere almost to the saturation point. Modern gardening finds excessive transpiration better secured by partial shade, and for room culture the atmosphere that human nature finds comfortable is found perfectly congenial to most plants, and far better to many than the moist atmosphere of the old-time greenhouses. The injury plants sometimes experience in rooms and house-conservatories comes rather from sulphurous gases escaping from gas-burners or heaters than from the lack of moisture in the atmosphere. Any atmosphere that is healthy for a human being is equally so for plants. As has been shown in a previous chapter, the action of both is reciprocal; the carbonic acid given off by human beings in the process of breathing just adds to the atmosphere what the plants take away; plants in return replace in the atmosphere the oxygen consumed by animal life. This nice balancing of powers refines a similar atmosphere for each, if the best conditions are to be reached. Plants grown in dwelling-houses thus add to the healthfulness of human beings. They do not give off much, if any, oxygen at night, but they pass what they receive from the room, adding nothing then to the volume. While, therefore, there is nothing at any time deleterious in plants even in sleeping-rooms, the general action of the foliage is to purify the atmosphere, while the ozone-producing property of plants in bloom tends to the destruction of matter injurious to human health.

Having treated of temperature, light, and moisture as they affect the atmosphere surrounding the stems and leaves of plants, we will offer a few suggestions on the same conditions as affecting the root.

Roots love darkness rather than light. They seem to feed on the nitrogen of the atmosphere, or on the nitrogeneous gases given off by the decaying organic matter of manures; but this matter seems to be made more advantageous to them by the presence of oxygen, hence the feeding-roots or fibres of plants keep as near the surface of the soil as they can consistently with their abhorrence of light. This is an important consideration in plant-growing, the best cultivators using every inducement to get the feeding-roots toward the surface. When a pot becomes full of roots, the plant has achieved for itself this condition in its best form, as all the ends of the fibres, which are the feeding portions, are around the inner surface of the pot, where, by the contraction and expansion during drying and receiving water, the air passes down more easily than through any other portion of the earth in the pot. Hence a plant that has the pot moderately well filled with roots is generally in better health than one only partly filled. A portion of the roots, however, do not care for getting near the reach of atmospheric air.

These are known as main, or tap-roots. They do not die annually, as the fibres do, but continue many years. These go down into the earth, and may be actually in water, not only without injury but often with positive benefit to the plant. To the larger roots water seems essential; to the fibres, moist air and no doubt water itself is in some degree acceptable; but the chief office that water performs in the food necessary for plant life is aiding in the supply of fresh air to the roots of plants. Besides aiding in the preparation of food, oxygen is a great foe to the lower order of fungi that preys on vegetable matter. A soil that does not admit air soon becomes what cultivators call "sour." In this condition minute moneds grow and feed on the tissues, when the leaves, deprived by the weakened power of the roots to procure food, take on a yellow cast. It is believed that the same cause—want of a full supply of oxygen—induces the vigorous growth of aspergillus, micrococcus, and other minute plants of a low organization, which are always found in increased quantities and in extreme vigor of development during the presence of epidemic diseases. Water introduces oxygen to the roots of plants by its superior weight. Penetrating into every little space and pore, it forces out completely every particle of air contained in the mass of earth. But as soon as the water sinks wholly away, passes wholly through the soil, the spaces are again open, and a new supply of oxygen follows where the water led.

It will thus be seen that a highly-saturated atmosphere—one that keeps plants from calling on the roots for moisture to supply the waste—is by no means one of the best for the healthy growth of plants; nor are those schemes which pack pots in wet or damp material, in order to prevent the soil from getting dry and thus save labor, much to be commended. A soil that permits the water to drain away with considerable ease, and in a day or two is again dry and asks for more water, is much better adapted to successful plant-growing than soil that, by labor-saving schemes, is prevented from getting but rarely dry.

Some very accurate experiments have recently been made in France and commented on by Duchartre, a famous vegetable physiologist. Wheat, rye, and oats were sown under equal conditions, and water supplied artificially. Taking 100 as the saturation point, the first set received 80, the second 60, the third 40, the fourth 30, the fifth 20, the sixth 10, and the seventh 5. Taking what should be a full crop to be represented by 100, the first equalled 19.16, the second 22.7, the third 21.7, the fourth 17.1, the fifth 14.6, the sixth 6.5, the seventh 0.1. Taking these figures as they stand, it would seem that over-watering is less likely to be injurious than a short supply,—and this may do for a general rule. But frequency of watering must not be confounded with over-watering. A well-drained soil in which water passes rapidly away never becomes saturated. A pot well drained may be watered daily to advantage, while one badly drained, and which will not permit the easy passage of water, may have the soil saturated by a watering of but once a week.

Sulphurous gases, as already noted, are very injurious to plants, but it has been noted that this violent element is much more injurious when it has access to the roots than to the leaves alone. A camellia has been confined for twenty-four hours exposed to an atmosphere of illuminating gas without any apparent injury, while trees that have their roots exposed to the gas in the earth from leaky city pipes generally die, and there are many cases known where in winter-time the gas from leaky city mains, prevented by frost from creeping through its usual course to the atmosphere, finds its way into greenhouses, permeates the earth in the flower-pot, and produces great destruction. Those who wish to pursue this study further may peruse with interest an interesting paper by B. A. Fahnestock in the *Proceedings of the American Philosophical Society.*

A mooted question with plant-growers is the advantage to be gained by using water warmer than that furnished from wells or rain-water cisterns. Those who have floral establishments and cannot arrange for warming water, but have to use it as naturally presented, believe it is of little use to warm it, as results seem to them every way satisfactory, and they refer to cases in forcing fruit where a grape-vine may have its roots in earth solidly frozen, or nearly so, while the branches are subjected to heat under glass that the roots are free from. There is no difficulty in getting fruits as early as seems desirable. Branches of vines have been taken into warmer houses, leaving others with the remaining branches in houses without any artificial heat. These branches, introduced to the warmer temperature, push into leaf and bear fruit apparently as well as if the whole plant with its roots had been equally warmed. Certainly this proves that warmth at the root is not essential to a growth of leaves or branches where the temperature of the atmosphere is sufficiently high. But wherever careful experiments have been made it is found that growth is accelerated by earth-warmth as well as a warm atmosphere, and this, indeed, is the foundation of what professional florists call "systems of bottom heat." For house or conservatory culture, wherever it is desirable to accelerate the flowering of plants, water of the temperature of seventy degrees will be found of much benefit.

Articles in which to grow plants may be ordinary flower-pots, vases, pans, shells, rustic baskets of wood or wire, or even blocks of trees, for there are plants known as epiphytes, of which the beautiful family of orchidæ furnish well-known examples, that grow better on such branches than in pots of ordinary sort. If attention has been paid to the preceding remarks, it will be evident that it will make but little difference in what a plant is grown so long as the soil will not dry too rapidly, nor hold water so that it shall not pass quickly away. The hole in the bottom of a flower-pot is to permit the rapid escape of water. We cannot grow plants in tin cans, bowls, or other articles of household use, simply because water cannot escape rapidly, indeed not at all. When plants are set in vessels of this character they are really growing in water, though, being filled with earth, the water may not be seen. The plants known as aquatics will grow in water, but these form a very small portion of what the cultivator desires, and these depend largely on the materials in the water for the means of existence. And there are sub-aquatics that succeed fairly well for a little time in water or wet soil, but require a larger situation for their complete or best development. The hyacinth blooms well in glasses of water in our rooms and greenhouses, but the bulb has to be grown in rich garden earth for a season, or even several seasons, before it will succeed in water as well as we usually find bulbs to do. And then it is well known that a hyacinth bulb, flowered in water one year, is almost useless another season. It gets from the water but little of the elements necessary to store food for future use. There is, indeed, no plant in general culture, except those known as aquatic, but which should have pots or vessels so arranged as to encourage water to pass away as rapidly as possible. Often holes are made at the sides near the bottom, as well as in the bottom itself, but if the flower-pot is properly made, there is seldom necessity for this. A first-class flower-pot should not have a perfectly flat bottom, but one slightly concave; the water passes more readily than when quite flat. Orchids, or other plants that particularly like an abundance of air at the roots, are often treated to pots that are purposely perforated, and it is said by good cultivators that many more plants would prefer these pots than many persons have any knowledge of. The ordinary clay flower-pots, being porous, permit much more moisture to evaporate than those which are glazed, or wooden boxes, hence there is not the same necessity to provide special avenues for the drainage of water as in other cases. Indeed, where pots are small and exposed to a drying atmosphere, many cultivators are indifferent whether their small pots admit of ready drainage or not. Plants that creep over the surface and do not send roots deep into the earth, such as lycopodiums, tradescantias, or spiderworts, marantas, or many ferns, must be provided with shallow pans. Ornamental pots, in which the ordinary flower-pot with the pan may be placed, are often employed, but these should have a stand at the bottom, so that after the plant has been watered the water may pass out wholly below the bottom of the pot holding the plant. Shells must have holes for the escape of water, though some arrangement should be provided for catching the fluid whenever the drainage through may prove annoying.

Where flower-pots have to be placed in situations in which the drainage would be found annoying, saucers may be used to great advantage. If the soil in the pot is so open that water will readily pass through to the saucer, no injury will result from a little water standing in the saucer: good will in many cases follow from such permission; but if the soil be closed and the roots weak, the water will rise in the earth by capillary attraction, and the earth become saturated, which we have already seen is injurious to the well-being of the growing plant. Long, narrow pots are often used for hyacinths and other bulbs that send their roots straight down into the earth. Flower-pots are now often made with square rims instead of round ones, as in general use in former years; this is simply a measure of economy. In packing away under the old system, one pot pressed into the other caused numbers to break. Under the modern plan, the pots rest under each other's shoulder and the pressure is avoided. Large pots have wires fastened around under the rims, to avoid the breakages which large masses of soil inside, pressing outward, often induce. Baskets for hanging plants should be made of galvanized wire to avoid rust, and blocks for orchideous plants selected from among the hard-wood trees, and if the truncheons have the rough bark on, so much the better.

All these vessels being provided with holes or passages for the rapid draining away of water, material must be provided to assist this operation. In all florists' establishments many pots get broken, and these are employed in this useful work. They are broken in pieces about the size of hickory-nuts,— large or smaller according to the size of the plants to be potted,—and a portion placed over the hole in the bottom of the pot. Over these broken pieces mats, sod, or any rough soil is placed. The object in using these broken pots or potsherds is to keep a vacuum into which the water drains slowly, and the mat or material is placed over to keep the earth from getting in the material, which would choke and destroy the vacuum. Broken bricks, gravel-stones, or any similar material will do where potsherds cannot be had.

The soil for potting should be almost dry, and the necessary material mixed well together. Until recently mixtures were made by means of a riddle, but of late years this has been abandoned by the ablest florists. It seems to destroy the turfy, spongy character that tends to keep the soil open and loose. The hands are employed to mix the material, or, if very turfy, the spade or trowel is used to chop the chunks apart.

In putting the plant in the pot the roots are kept as near the surface as possible, and when the dry earth is put in it is rammed in with a thick piece of wood, or anything that is suitable for ramming, as hard as it is possible to ram it. If the soil is as dry as it ought to be, the hard ramming pulverizes the soil and makes the whole a much more porous mass than a tight pressing would. If the soil be damp, heavy ramming or pressing will have the contrary effect. The pot containing the plant should never be larger than is necessary to comfortably contain the roots. Some good cultivators fill the pots pretty full, but it is best to leave at least a quarter of an inch for water. Basket plants usually like a good mixture of moist or spongy material, packed in pretty tight, as being exposed to the atmosphere on all sides, it is an extra provision against drying out. Orchids are fastened to blocks by wires, and most usually introduced to furnish a little moisture at the start, but as soon as the new growth of roots attach themselves to the block they need no other covering. Moss has been used instead of soil for potting. Bone-dust or some other fertilizer is added, and the whole mass of material packed in very tightly about the plants. Some excellent results have been obtained by the use of moss in this way.

After plants have been potted they usually receive a thorough soaking of water, and, if the potted plant has many leaves and is likely to wilt, it is placed in a dark place, as dark as possible, in order to check transpiration till the roots are able to help the plant to some moisture. As already noticed, on first potting the plant should be placed in as small a pot as the roots will go in, but as soon as the roots appear on the outside of the ball, near the inner edge of the pot, in any large numbers, it is shifted to a larger one, and again shifted as it needs. Good cultivators often shift a plant several times in a single season, and a number of times when it is desirable to grow some plants to great perfection. To ascertain whether a plant needs potting, it is turned upside down, the plant between the fingers, and the edge of the pot tapped against a wooden bench. The plant with its ball falls out, and the pot is held in the right hand. If the pot is very full of roots the pot is held fast, even though it gets a rough notice to let go; in these cases the ball should be thoroughly soaked with water first, then it slips out easily. Large plants lifted from the ground for potting often wilt badly, even though carefully moved and kept in moist, cool, and shady places. To lessen this as much as possible, some of the older leaves are taken off, or the branches may be thinned out; but if even these precautions are not likely to be sufficient, the young and tender portions of the stock, that would transpire the most heavily, are shortened back as far as it seems likely to serve the object we have in view. Plants under these circumstances are like cuttings; and frequently we have to take off all the leaves permanently in order to check the escape of moisture till the roots are formed. Striking cuttings is not the mysterious art it used to be. When a piece of a plant is put in the earth without roots, its vital power is at a low ebb. It has to put forth all its energies to save itself. In this condition low forms of fungi, that are ever on the alert to profit by low vital conditions, attack and often destroy the cuttings. Fungus attacks, indeed, are the cause of almost all failures to make cuttings grow. Since this has been discovered, the effort is to keep fungus away. Fungus cannot work well under water; hence, if cuttings are placed in saucers of sand full of water, and given enough heat to induce heat-growth, they nearly always grow. As soon as they root, however, they must be transferred to earth potted, as already noted. Cuttings in pots of earth should be kept cool till they show a disposition to grow; but, though cool, the temperature should be above the dew-point, as that is particularly favorable to fungus-growth inimical to insects. It is often desirable to raise seeds in pots. If fine, they should be placed very near the surface, and sometimes glass may be placed over for a short time in order to preserve a uniform degree of moisture without much watering, which is very much against success. Seeds love darkness during germination, but as soon as activity begins they must have light in order to place the growing plants. The general rule is to pot seedlings as soon as they make one or two rough leaves, as they are called; that is, the leaves immediately succeeding the seed-leaves. They must be watered immediately after the operation, as wilting in a young seedling is often fatal.

Much of the pleasure of plant-growing depends on training. An unshapely plant is seldom a "thing of beauty," no matter how healthy it may be. Leaves and growing branches have an attraction for light,—hence plants are liable to get one-sided. Frequent turning is an advantage. Theoretically, frequent turning is a disadvantage, but the injury is slight, and the greater uniformity in the plant compensation in full.

Tall, "leggy" plants are often undesirable. To avoid this, the central bud of the young seedling or cutting is taken out. This causes a number of side-shoots instead of one leader. When these grow a few inches they are again pinched back, if a still more bushy plant is desirable. This pinching back has to be done at an early stage of growth, or it interferes with the proper blooming of a plant. If, for instance, the plant in question be a chrysanthemum or a bouvardia, which flowers in early winter, the cutting is rooted in about February or March. About the 1st of May it will have its first pinchings, and about the 1st of June the second. If it were pinched again about the 1st of July the plant would be still more bushy, but the flowers would be very small. In all cases pinching, to make plants bushy, is at the expense of the size of the flower. We sacrifice a little of this to make a bushy plant, but it is so little as not to be a great disadvantage. A frequent repetition of the operation would, however, show the injury to be material. To assist in obtaining a good form, light painted stakes are used. No more than absolutely required should be used, and no longer retained than necessary to direct the twig in the way it should go. Exhibition plants are often rendered repulsive by the number of training stalks about them. In tying, a twist is made around the stake. This prevents the tying material from slipping down, and permits a large loop around the twig or branch, so that no injury to the branch results. Some plants show to best advantage when trained on flat trellises. These may be made neatly of small stakes or galvanized wire. Some plants that have a somewhat drooping habit of growth or inflorescence are best trained to a single stem in the centre of the pot. The fuchsia or the lantana are much prettier when trained in this style.

Though very much of the pleasure of plant-growing depends on the art of training the plants properly, it is an art almost wholly overlooked by writers on floriculture, and seldom put into practice by cultivators generally.

A very interesting part of flower-growing, and which may fairly be treated of under the head of potting, is raising new varieties from seed. Nearly all the beautiful varieties known as florists' flowers have been raised artificially. Geraniums, fuchsias, coleus, and many things in common cultivation are very different from what they were when fresh from the hand of nature. In nature plants vary, but the varieties do not get a chance for perpetuation. Of the thousands of seeds wild plants produce, only a few develop into perfect plants again. Thus a variation has many more chances of an early disappearance than of persistence. But when a variation strikes the eye of the cultivator, the seeds are saved, and thus the departure becomes hereditary. This is called selection. Nature is simply assisted to perpetuate the variations she herself makes. In this alone consists the florist's art. When, therefore, we desire to get new varieties, all we have to do is to look among the seedlings for any marked forms or variations, and save the seed. From seedlings of these, again save from the striking departures. In time, forms are raised very different from the original parent. This is the slower method. A more rapid is by crossing.

We may have a white and a red zonale pelargonium, or geranium, as they are commonly called. As soon as the flower opens, we take the pollen and place it over the stigma of the white,—the stigma being the extreme central portion of the flower. Seeds resulting from this operation will have flowers varying between white and red. To make the operation as secure as we wish it, care must be taken to apply the pollen-dust to the stigma before it has had any chance to receive its own. To make this secure, some florists open the flower before it expands naturally, and take off the anthers,— the parts producing the pollen before they mature. Then they wait a day or two for the stigma to mature before applying the pollen from the other flower, or, if applying the pollen at once after taking off the anthers, they apply more pollen of the kind a few days after.

The chief discouragements in plant-growing come from the perpetual war on insects one has to wage. The plant-grower is never at rest. Though the whole crop of insect enemies be destroyed, their eggs are usually secure; a light frost may destroy the insect, but the egg goes through the lowest temperature, and hatches whenever a little warmer weather comes, so that continual watchfulness is essential. Many are very small, or are in some way concealed, and often they do great damage before their presence is known. The good plant-grower should have a pocket-lens, and be continually on the alert to discover their first appearance. When the eye becomes practised, the presence of insects is readily detected. It may be a light yellow or gray streak on the leaf, or the leaf may slightly curl,—anything, indeed, out of the normal appearance of a leaf or stem will create suspicion that something is wrong, and generally the wrong is to be referred to an insect or to a fungus. The two most common insects on pot-plants are the green fly, a species of aphis, and the red spider, the latter so called because it belongs to the same general order as the common spider, though it feeds on plants and is not carnivorous. Like ordinary spiders, too, they form a web, but the web is not used except to travel on.

The green fly usually congregates at the ends of the growing stems and leaves, the pieces of which it sucks for a living. They are readily destroyed by spraying with water heated to about 130°. When it is inconvenient to spray, as is often the case when plants are grown in the house, a tub of water tested by a thermometer to 130° may be placed near the plants, and the plant, inverted in the hand, may be dipped for an instant in the water. Tobacco-water is sometimes used, warmed to the same temperature. The leaf-stalks of the tobacco obtained from cigar-makers are steeped in water, a pound of stems to a gallon of water being used. Tobacco-smoke is the most successful where it can be used, as in a whole greenhouse, or under a barrel. A little paper or wood is used to start a fire in some old vessel, moistened tobacco-stalks placed over, and then left to burn out. Those who may desire neater utensils will find many styles of fumigators in those establishments that keep florists' supplies. Where plants are trained over walls or in rooms, and it is not convenient to take them down to dip in liquid or destroy by tobacco-smoke, fine powder of tobacco sprinkled over the damp places is used to good advantage.

The red spider is one of the worst pests to the plant-grower. The pocket-lens should be always in use to detect its presence. It does not like moisture, hence it is not found to be troublesome where plants often can be syringed. The fumes from very warm sulphur also annoy the insect. Hence, florists who have large greenhouses wash hot-water or steam-pipes with sulphur, or place sulphur on a piece of slate in the hot sun. But if sulphur ignites it makes sulphuric acid, which is extremely injurious to vegetation. Quite a number of washes are offered as good against red spider and other insects, the exact ingredients of which are not made public. Fir-tree oil is one of these.

The thrip is perhaps the next in order of troublesome insects. It is a small, narrow, black or brown insect, and seems to prefer plants with a firm texture of leaves. The azalea, camellia, and ferns with heavy fronds are illustrations. It is very rapid in its movements, and skips effectively when disturbed. Its presence is not often known till the numerous whitish lines among the green are observed. Tobacco-smoke and tobacco-infusions are good when the insect can be made to endure them, but they fall to the ground frequently when the smoke begins to annoy them, and get up again when the smoke is gone. Dipping in water at 130° is the best remedy when it can be done. There is a species of this insect very troublesome to the carnation-grower, known in professional life as the "twitters."

Scale insects are of several genera. Some are round, others shell-like, and others of various forms and sizes. They are frequently on the orange, lemon, oleander, some ferns, camellias, and many others. These are all killed by the warm-water treatment. Whale-oil soap is also useful, applied with a sponge or brush. Vegetable oils have been used to advantage, and some have had success with diluted alcohol.

The mealy bug is a persevering enemy of the plant-grower. Though one may go over a plant and kill every one, more will soon appear, from minute eggs that were overlooked. Kerosene emulsion is best for this,—about a gallon of kerosene and about a half-gallon of cow's milk with it, poured in gradually and stirred till it becomes like thin butter. Condensed milk with half its bulk of water will do, if cow's milk cannot be obtained. This is also useful against other insects as well as the mealy bug.

There are not many other insects likely to prove troublesome to the plant-grower. Sometimes the blue woolly aphis is troublesome at the roots of plants, but water at about 150° destroys them and does not hurt the plant. In like manner ants, worms, wood-lice, wireworms, cutworms, or similar pests may be hastened away. For these lime-water is often found effectual. A lump of lime is placed in a vessel of water, which is left undisturbed for a day or so. Only the clear liquid is used. Wood-lice and slugs are often troublesome, but these are easily trapped; a piece of apple or boiled potato or other similar thing is placed near their haunts, and covered to keep dry and dark. They will collect here, and will be easily caught and destroyed. In large places where roses are forced into bloom in the winter, there has been recently found a rose beetle named by entomologists Aramigus Fulleri. It is a small brown beetle, rather smaller than the common rose "bug" or beetle of our gardens in early summer. It is injurious by feeding on the leaves, and by the larvæ feeding on the roots. The rose-growers watch and catch by hand and destroy the beetles, which so far is the only remedy known.

Rusts, mildews, and moneds, going generally under the name of microscopic fungi, are great foes of the plant-grower. They were formerly considered merely as the consequence of some disease; now they are well understood to cause some diseases, and have therefore an increased importance. A plant may have, by bad treatment or other causes, a low vital power, but it would continue to do comparatively well for a long time only for these minute enemies. Their attacks are then successful. To this extent they may be the cause of disease. But that they attack, injure, and kill sometimes, even when plants are in their normal healthful condition, is now conceded. The worst and most troublesome form at the present time is known as the verbena rust. This blackens and curls the opening leaves as they grow, and the plant finally succumbs. It attacks heliotrope, tomatoes, and many other plants. It probably belongs to the same class of minute fungus-plants that is so destructive to the potato-plant and known as perenospora. Some have found minute insects in connection with this trouble so far as the verbena is concerned, and have thought they may be the actual cause of the trouble.

The rose mildew is also a serious trouble with rose-growers. The growing leaves are often whitened as with powder. Some varieties are more liable to it than others, and this is taken as evidence that it follows a weakened vital power. Strong, robust growers are usually free from it. Still, it can be kept from growing and spreading even on plants of low vitality by good precautions. The roots have to be kept in good condition by good drainage, good healthy soil, and not suffered to get too low a temperature by cold weather. Cold draughts of air are also to be guarded against, and sudden changes from a dry to moist air or a high to low temperature. Indeed, where a regularly high temperature both for root and branch is maintained, mildew is seldom troublesome. There are other forms of fungus attacks that have troubled rose-growers of later years,—one known as the black leaf fungus, and one the black spot on the stem. But these are not found to be very annoying until the plants are over two years old. Without troubling themselves, therefore, with the causes or cures, the florists replace with growing plants every year or so. Sulphur and hot water are the only two remedies known for mildew so far. A dusting of the leaves affected with sulphur often stops the spread, and in plant-houses it is placed on plates where the sun or warm flues can make some vapor from it. Syringing of hot water also checks its growth. Carnations and many other plants suffer at times from a white cobweb-like fungus at the root. Hot water at 150°, with sulphur, is a sure remedy, unless the fungus has gone so far as to cause an actual decay of the main roots, which in carnations it often does before it is suspected.

In almost all houses warmed by modern contrivances, sanitary science complains of the aridity of the atmosphere. Attempts have been made to remedy this by having evaporators connected with cellar heaters. Hygrometers show little advantage from these contrivances, the high temperature at which the water evaporates probably carrying the highly-rarefied vapor away with the waste heat, which must always escape in order to secure circulation. But in living plants we have an admirable arrangement for furnishing the atmosphere of rooms with moisture at a comparatively low temperature, as the whole of their active life is spent in transmitting moisture, which they draw from the soil by means of their roots, through their leaves into the atmosphere. A flower-pot with earth saturated with moisture will be damp after several days; but if a vigorous plant be growing therein, the moisture will be sucked out and transmitted to the air in the room in a few hours. This illustrates the value of plants in softening the rigors of a dry atmosphere. For this purpose plants with thin leaves are preferable to those with thick leaves,—thick leaves generally being thick in order to prevent the escape of their moisture. A cactus has an epidermis so thick that it transpires but little. It is thus suited to dry deserts, and places where there is little rain. It will retain its moisture for months, because none escapes through the skin. In a room the wax-plant will behave much in the same way. It requires water less freely than most broad-leaved plants. A camellia needs more water than a wax-plant, but less than the azalea, and this again less than the geranium, for, though the leaves are thin the stems are woody. In brief, the thinner the leaves the more water they waste, if waste it may be called. This is additional advantage of great importance to the sanitary influences plants are known to exercise upon the atmosphere.

But the purifying influence of plants is not confined to the leaves alone, as was formerly supposed. It is but recently that blossoms, flowers themselves, are known as ozone-producers, and in this way present us with new reasons for their existence on the earth. Until this fact was discovered, their actual use in the economy of nature was but imperfectly understood. Poets sang praises to the loveliness of flowers, and the devout gave thanks that they were made to enjoy a world which flowers had rendered so beautiful. Those who looked deeper into the philosophy of nature saw in the colors of flowers an attraction to insects, and insects rendered service by carrying pollen from strange flowers, thus aiding cross-fertilization, which was believed to be a benefit to the race. And the odors,—the sweet emanations from the flowers,—these also were mere superabundancies to give additional attraction to the insect visitors. It is remarkable that any other use for beautiful flowers should have been so long unsuspected, as it is clear in every department of nature beings are made to contribute something to the general good that may be in no way related to their individual interests. Not only are the gay and gaudy blossoms throwing their continual efforts into the general welfare, but myriads of inconspicuous flowers such as grasses are perpetually employed in this purifying process.

These discoveries of later years give a new interest to the window-gardener. He or she desires not only to know how to grow plants, but to have plants that will be continually in flower. He will be anxious to secure not merely a "greenery," as window-gardening has been termed, but a floral bower, as well as the luxuries which healthful foliage always affords. Flowers as well as plants thus become a necessity of modern times.

All books on window-gardening contend that if we would have plants to bloom, a south, southeast, or southwest aspect is indispensable. This is far from the fact. We may have flowers in any window that has a fair share of light, but we must select the plants favorable in each case. Those kinds which flower on the new growth, such as all annuals, and fuchsias, geraniums, roses, carnations, and similar plants, must have sunlight to do well. These are plants that leave flowering as the last stage of growth. But there is a large class of plants that only make flower-buds before they go to rest, and then make flowering the first operation under the new start in growth the following season. All of this class will flower as well in a room with light, though wholly deprived of sun, as in the best southern aspect. Hyacinths, tulips, crocus, Chinese primroses, dandelions, violets, cyclamens, and numerous others are of this class. True, they have to form their buds under full sunlight the season before, but as most window-gardeners in America have their plants in the open air during summer and until late in autumn, this is readily accomplished. Even the pretty calla lily, or Richardia Ethiopica, as botanists call it, will flower in a room deprived of direct sunlight if it has been grown in the full sunlight the autumn before. It is hardly worth while in a chapter of this kind to give lists of plants, because frequently they are difficult to obtain, and often others quite as good as those recommended may be obtained from friends or neighboring florists. In order, however, that the reader may understand the class we mean when we say plants which perfect their buds the fall before, we may give, in addition to those already named, camellia, azalea, periwinkle, deutzia, narcissus, amaryllis, and most bulbs.

There are, however, some plants that flower towards the end of their young growth, and which would bloom fairly well in partial shade. Among these are oranges and lemons. Begonias, a very numerous family, having some four hundred species in a wild state, would afford a full window-full in themselves. Lily of the valley, jasmine, ivy geranium, Haytien myrtle, tradescantia, or spiderwort, commelyna, Kenilworth ivy, and saxifrage.

Those which flower as they grow must, however, generally have sunlight in order to get the best effects from them. This is a very large class, of which in illustration the following may be named as adapted to window-culture: geraniums, or pelargoniums, chrysanthemums, roses, cactuses, mesembryanthemums, and many succulents; but these, above all, must have the full sun: fuchsias, mignonette, pansies, mimulus, or monkey-flowers, heliotrope, oleander, rose geraniums, and a number of other Cape species, such as apple-scented pepper, nutmeg, and the like, all of which like full sun, musk-plants, mahernia, abutilon, and others.

There are, however, famous window-plants that cannot be dispensed with, though grown for their foliage alone. The parlor ivy, Senecio scandens and S. macroglossa, and the good old stand-by, the English ivy, with its numerous varieties, are indispensable. The india-rubber, Ficus elastica, wax-plant, Hoya carnosa, and the very large family of ferns and lycopodiums, must also have a place.

If there be an abundance of space, plenty of bright light, and we can make sure of victory in the struggle with red spider and determined foes in the insect world, we may undertake nasturtiums, maurantias, petunias, lobelias, balsams, pansies, and such like. These flower towards spring, and carry our window-gardening into the season when the open air successfully competes with our window-work. Those, however, who have only small city yards and have their chief flower-gardens on roofs, balconies, or even window-sills, will find these plants just the things to help them to blossoms all the year round.

How to keep out the frost, or rather to keep up the heat, so as to have blooming plants all the winter through, is often a puzzle with many. But much of this anxiety might be avoided by selecting plants according to the heat that we can afford them. There are a large number of wild-flowers, perfectly hardy, that bloom almost before the frost is gone, that would do perfectly well for rooms in which little or no fire is kept. These come forward with so little heat that there would be no trouble in having them blossom six weeks or two months before they appeared in the open air. The dandelion and the buttercup, violets, English primroses, and pansies are of this class. There are also dwarf evergreens, such as mahonia, perfectly hardy, and which flower with very little warmth, that would be very desirable. The Japan Euonymus, though not flowering, is a very pretty evergreen for cold-room culture.

It is, however, in the parlor, dining-room, and the bedroom, where the temperature is usually above 60°, that we want blooming plants; and even plants naturally hardy, or nearly so, when forced into vigorous growth, must have protection from low temperature and from frost. The worst foe in these cases is illuminating gas; where the pressure on the gas is great, some will escape burning and get into the room. Much of the trouble usually referred to "the dry air from the heater" really comes from this, and even when the heater is responsible it is rather sulphurous vapor than the dryness of the "heat" that is responsible. Hence all arrangements for warming plant-rooms by either gas-jets or from coal-furnaces are dangerous. Where wood stoves, coke, or coal-oil arrangements can be introduced there is no trouble in growing window-plants. Where we are perfectly sure no coal-gas will get in from the heater in the cellar, we are also safe against danger. It is usually in the night-time that plants suffer from these causes. Dampers are down, or the fires are banked up for the night, and then with scarcely any draft the gases escape into the atmosphere instead of going into the smoke-flue, or, the gas being turned down low, aids in the escape of a portion unconsumed. Where there is a certainty of enough heat being preserved in a portion of the room where the plants are, they may be preserved against this danger by having curtains drawn across. This is often adopted where plants are grown in bay-windows. Close-fitting shutters against the glass keep out the frost, and curtains drawn against the wall-line on the inner side of the bay projection together keep the plants sound and safe against frost from without or gas within.

To get at the windows for closing shutters or the other work, the stages, stands, boxes, or vases in which plants are grown, or in which they are placed, should be easily movable, and in most cases this will be easily accomplished by having castors placed beneath. Exact designs for stands or tables are of little use. These have to be suited to the room or to one's conveniences in the room. Where there is a bay-window, however, a very pretty flower-stand is a cone made of two, three, or more series of shelves, the upper or terminal circle being only large enough for a single pot. This should be set on castors so as to easily revolve, when each day, or twice each day, the whole mass may be turned a little towards the light. Every few days, therefore, every plant gets a full share of the light, without having to spend its own energies in turning to get it. This low, conical stage permits of flowers almost from the ground, and admits of arches over, formed of English ivy, parlor ivy, or some similar twining or trailing plant, which adds much to the interest of the room. Another advantage of this circular stage is that it permits of other small stands and brackets against the wall, and facing the stage, which, by breaking up the space into smaller sections, adds to its apparent extent, besides giving light by which more plants can be grown than when all are in one solid block. Wire stages, galvanized, of course, to prevent rust, are sometimes used, but unless very strongly made, which they seldom are, they are not able to bear the weight, and soon get disturbed, or otherwise lose favor. Wood, made as light as possible, is best. Arrangements must be made to catch the waste water; saucers under each pot give the best safeguard. Oilcloth, zinc, or painted tin, slightly elevated in parts and so placed on the ground that all the drip will run into one point, where it collects in a vessel, has been employed. Some good housekeepers, who know just how much water to give plants without waste, simply drop a piece of old burlap under the plants to catch what may accidentally fall. Light galvanized wire trellises are very useful around and over windows, up corners, and over doors where there is some light, in order to train ivy and other climbing plants. It is best, however, to have the wires so that they can be easily drawn out from the plants, as it is often desirable to do so, in order that the vines may be taken down and dipped in warm water to destroy insects, or perhaps to get at the wall to clean and paint, or for other causes. Indeed, in order to keep absolute control of any event of this character, the good window-gardener seldom permits the vine to twine in its own wilful way among the meshes of the wire trellis, but ties the young growth along on the front face of the trellis as it grows.

Then by cutting the tying material the vine can at any time be easily taken down.

Hanging baskets, of course, add naturally to the interest of window-culture. Wire baskets, rustic baskets formed of roots or knotty branches, shells, cocoanut-shells with holes or projections to allow of ferns or other plants to protrude along the whole surface, give great variety. In these days much need not be said in a chapter of this character on the matter of styles, as every large florist's catalogue is filled with them. In a general way we may say that some of these very pretty things as offered are by no means the best to grow plants, and after some time become dirty and shabby; and frequently the commonest things, cheaply made by oneself or those around, will have more lasting beauty than the best model from a fancy store.

Plant-cases are useful for ferns or such plants as desire a very close and moist atmosphere. The object of this chapter is to encourage chiefly the use of plants that produce flowers as room ornaments; but where it is desirable to grow plants in cases, it may be well to note that it is not well to have the glass perfectly close, because moisture condenses on the inside of the glass, which is, in many respects, undesirable. It is better for many reasons that two portions of the glass case be made to open or tilt, in order that the plants may be handled or examined easily if necessary, in such cases it will be easy to have the opening portion ajar at times.

Aquariums are interesting when properly understood and well cared for. The same principle prevails under water as in the atmosphere, that it requires a balance of plant and of animal life to lead to health. Water in which are only plants soon becomes green and unpleasant to look at, while water in which there are no plants *will not* support fish or other living creatures. The oxygen which plants expire is just what the fish require for support, while the carbonic acid the fish exhale goes towards the support of the plants. It is this principle that lies at the bottom of successful aquarium management. Fish or other living creatures and plants must go together. It, however, requires much care and patience to be very successful. The glass must be kept clean to look neat. The earth in which the plants are to grow must have stones or something like this packed around, to keep the fish from keeping it stirred up. Very often the fish will so eat or worry the water-plants that they make only a feeble growth. In such cases it is best to have the water-plants in a pot in the centre of the aquarium, and then to have a screen of galvanized wire surrounding pot and plants extending up through the water, and through which only the smallest fish can enter. Very few persons, however, continue long to take pleasure in room aquariums, chiefly because in spite of the best of care fish become diseased and die, when, as already noted, the water smells disagreeable and interest in the affair ceases.

It is customary to tell those who would be perfect in cultivating window-plants that they cannot work without tools, and that they ought to have half-leather gloves for keeping the hands clean, a pair of scissors, penknife, light trowel, water-pot with a spout so small that the water will not come out very rapidly in watering, small pots, and there should be a movable section of small spout, so as to make it larger when desirable to get at plants some distance from the manipulator. A small syringe, a sprayer, and a pocket-lens to look after disease or insects, as well as to examine the more minute parts of flowers and plants, in which often lie a great deal of interest; but the successful window-gardener is, after all, usually born and not made. We have endeavored only to lay down several principles, and those who will succeed must fill up the details in order to become professors of the art.

A greenhouse is the place wholly given up to the growth of plants. A conservatory, in the original use of the term, is a greenhouse-like structure, usually attached to the dwelling, into which plants are taken when in bloom, to be returned to the greenhouse when out of flower. The terms are much mixed in these modern times; small greenhouses when attached to dwellings being often termed conservatories.

Wherever able to afford the luxury, there is nothing more desirable than to have both of them. Then one of the objects of this work—which is to encourage the use of plants in flower about our home—would be more readily attained. It is very desirable for many reasons to have the two separate. When the greenhouse is separate from the dwelling there is no trouble about the heating as there is in the dwelling, and all the dust and dirt and confusion incident to cleaning wholly avoided. When comparatively no trouble to grow plants in a house that is wholly theirs, it requires much art, skill, and good judgment to grow plants in rooms together with ourselves. Now, the conservatory is a much more simple affair than a greenhouse. The provision for abundant light so necessary for the latter is not essential here; indeed, flowers stay longer in bloom and are in every way more satisfactory when in partial shade than when in the full sun. Again, a comparatively low temperature is much more favorable for keeping flowers a long time in bloom, and a temperature of about 55° is all that a good conservatory requires.

Conservatories are more favorable for ornamentation than mere greenhouses, where plants have to be grown as well as flowered. They may be quite lofty, and this will give room for a few plants of temperate regions that flower in winter to remain the whole winter there. The Australian acacias are of this class; they grow from five to ten or twenty feet high, and from late winter to spring give forth a profusion of gay yellow and often sweet flowers, that give a great charm to all the rest. Oranges, lemons, and similar plants in large pots or tubs may often be wintered in the lofty conservatory, while the smaller plants only may be introduced from the greenhouse from time to time. The conservatory is always an attachment to the dwelling-house, and is usually made in connection with the dining-room. In modern times, when cut flowers and even living plants are essential ornaments to a meal-table, we can well understand the additional charm that a whole vista of flowering plants gives.

Small conservatories give but little trouble in the way of heating. The roof may be of thick ground glass, and so tightly set that no heat can escape. The side-lights may be of double sashes, and, if there is a storm-door to the exit, the interior will be nearly frost-proof. An arrangement to burn a few coal-oil lamps during cold nights, or a coke stove, or even in many cases the leaving open of the door connecting with the retiring-room, will be a sufficient protection against frost.

If more pretentious conservatories are desirable, some neat hot-water arrangement will be necessary. Where dwelling-houses are heated by steam,—and the number of these are continuously increasing,—a radiator here and there can be very easily introduced. It is indeed much in favor of heating any dwelling by steam, that it overcomes much of the difficulty usually found in window- or house-gardening. In proportion as steam-heating is cheapened and made suitable for even small dwellings, will houses with flowers increase and attract. Even a greenhouse wholly separated from the dwelling may be heated by a connection with the same apparatus when the dwelling is heated by steam.

Where the plant-room is to be both greenhouse and conservatory, as with a majority of our readers such will likely be the case, some care will be required to provide light, warmth, and ventilation. It must not be forgotten that direct sunlight is necessary to secure the best efforts from growing plants for the production of flowers, hence the scope of the glass, the aspect, and other considerations must have reference to this fact. Plants also love to be as near the glass as possible; they are liable to be drawn and spindly when grown at a distance away. Only ferns, and those known as leaf-plants, do well at distances away. Whatever design is adopted, these facts must be kept in view. At one time much of the usefulness of a plant-house was lost through the supposed necessity of elaborate schemes for ventilation. Usually, quite enough air will find its way into a greenhouse for the successful growth of plants. The ventilation should be arranged chiefly with the view of permitting the lowering of the temperature on warm days; about seventy degrees is quite high enough for a successful conservatory.

The arrangement of the conservatory, or combined greenhouse and conservatory, will depend wholly on the design and the situation. They are often square in their ground outline, or are a parallelogram, or a combination of lines and curves. If ferns, rockeries, or fountains can be introduced, the design may be made to conform to the objects. Usually, however, the structure is built from the architect's plans, without any consultation with the plant-cultivator, simply because it enters into some ornamental design for the whole dwelling, and without the slightest reference to the main object for which the conservatory is built. Numbers of such affairs may be seen in our country. Plants cannot be grown in them; they are no permanent attraction, and too often prove but eye-sores or nuisances. Plans are also frequently furnished, by even good garden architects, of structures that have proved acceptable in some localities, that are of no use in another. It is, in brief, scarcely possible to offer any plans that will be just suited to a conservatory or attached greenhouse. The only safe way is to bear in mind the general principles noted for the successful growth, protection, and preservation of plants, and then see that the architect's plans of the building are in harmony with the dwelling and also in harmony with these general principles.

It is altogether different with greenhouse buildings; these, being separate from the dwelling, stand wholly on their own requirements. The design must be wholly subordinate to the great object, namely, the growth of plants. But even here the architect of the dwelling, who knows nothing of plant growth, is called in, and the end may be a beautiful but nearly useless structure. Our object is to get plenty of blooming plants at all times, and bright sunlight in winter is a great aid. Hence a steep pitch that permits the sun to send its rays directly against it is found much better than a flatter roof, which may admit plenty of light but not direct sunlight. The best angle will be one of forty-five degrees. Houses are often of a less steep slope than this. For the same reason it is best to have some perpendicular side sash, as the morning sun through these is very favorable to the production of flowers. As already noted, elaborate schemes for ventilation are not thought of as much consequence as formerly, but provision must be made for opening when the temperature rises above 70° or 80°. For this reason framed sash are not in as general use as formerly. These were to slide down. Now light bars are set in from the sills to the ridge-pole the width of the panes, and the glass set in them. Schemes for avoiding the use of putty are numerous in these days. In our climate putty often cracks, separates from the wood, makes a leaky house, and is annoying when repairs are made.

The upright or slide glasses are, however, puttied, as the weather does not raise the same objections here. This style of building is called the "fixed-roof" system. The arrangement of the inside may vary with the taste of the owner, but he must never forget that the plants love to be as near the glass as possible, desire as much sunlight as possible, must have as many of the sides of each plant exposed to the light as possible, and yet must be convenient to be easily seen and handled. Houses may be of a single style; that is to say, a single line of glass inclining from a back wall, or a double span, in which the glass slopes both ways, with a ridge-pole in the centre of the house. The former is old-fashioned, but winter-flowering plants love them very much. They are easily warmed and cost but little, and are easily managed. Sloping shelves are placed under the glass till they come down to a line about three feet from the floor, then there is a narrow path, and on the other side near the upright sash another table. If the house be a double span, this arrangement of course continues all round it.

The greatest study comes from heating the greenhouses. A large number of plants do not require a temperature of over 55° in order to bloom freely during winter. A house suited to this is called a greenhouse. One that has plants requiring 70° or 80° to grow well or flower the plants is called a hot-house. These are again subdivided among hot-house plants,— for instance, there may be the palm-house or the orchid-house. Those who desire simply plenty of blooming plants in the winter to take to the dwelling-house, or even to enjoy in the greenhouse itself, do not need very elaborate systems of heating. It is only when houses are required on an extensive scale that it is particularly desirable to have expensive arrangements for hot water or steam. Very well made smoke-rooms of fire-brick flue-pipe, if seamed from cracking, can be carried under the stage. The flues must be kept as much from the earth as possible, or the heat will be absorbed and dampness obstruct draught. Wherever a flue can be carried round and back, so that the chimney is right over the furnace, there is seldom much trouble from bad draught. The fire warms the chimney, and that induces draught. Wherever a little more expense is no great object hot-water pipes are much better, because the pipes take so little room, can be taken where flues cannot, and are much better and prettier every way.

Orchid-houses, rose-houses, and many houses in which specialties are wholly grown, give a great deal of pleasure to the flower-lover, but these are only built when one has already some experience. We design here to give but the elementary knowledge that will place the would-be cultivator on the starting-track. Our task would not be complete without a few suggestions on the growth of flowers in the open air. When nature furnishes the exhalations from health-giving blossoms everywhere about us, instead of wafting it on the breezes that have to bear their burdens from flowery regions while we are in charge of the ice-king, there is less sanitary reason for flower-culture than during the winter season. But garden art and the culture of flowers in rooms and under glass are so closely connected that our chapter would not be complete without a few words on out-door gardening.

The outer walls of a dwelling may be made a bower of plants in bloom nearly the whole year. It is not well to have the plants attached to the building, but on trellises, so that in the event of painting or repairs being required they can be taken down and set up again without much injury. The best material for trellises is galvanized wire. If the wall be stone, holes may be drilled, wooden pegs be solidly driven in, and then iron pegs about as thick as lead-pencils driven in so as to project four or six inches from the wall, or the ends of these iron pegs are eyes to which the wires forming the trellises are to be attached. These can be placed at bottom, top, and sides of the house, so as to make a net-work with meshes about a foot or so square. If the house be frame the pegs may be screwed in. On this frame the plants are framed. Trained against these, Chimonanthus fragrans, Forsythia suspensa, and Jasminum multiflorum will be in bloom long before the frost is gone. Akebia quinata immediately follows. Honeysuckles come directly after, then roses, then sweet clematis, and then the large flowering clematis and the Japan honeysuckle keep up the succession till the autumn frosts appear. These will mostly grow mixed together, so that on the same piece of wall there will be flowers the whole season through. There are a number of plants that will cling directly to the wall without any trellis. For instance, the American and Japan ampelopsis, the trumpet-vine, the Japan and American climbing hydrangeas, eunonymus, and the numerous varieties of English ivy. This is nearly the full list, and therefore does not afford the rich variety a trellis gives. Some have thought such clinging vines keep the walls damp. But this is a mistake, unless some of the branches are permitted to obstruct the gutters or choke the conduits. They rather keep the walls dry: the numerous rootlets by which they cling absorb moisture. The dryest walls in the world are the walls of the old ivy-covered ruins in the moist climate of Northern Europe. Where walls are very smooth the evergreen or English ivy does not adhere well, but if the American ampelopsis or trumpet are planted with it, the extra assistance enables it to hold.

Beds of hardy herbaceous plants and hardy annuals are particularly desirable for furnishing a great variety of forms during every season of the year.

Since what is known as the bedding or massing system has come into vogue, there has been found a great want of flowering plants in most gardens. These beds are found worthy of plants with colored leaves, such as coleus or achyranthus, or with numerous varieties of geraniums, petunias, or similar well-known plants. In these fashionable gardens hardly any place has been left for the great variety of flowering plants old-fashioned gardens once had. But their culture should be encouraged. There is nothing better for these than long, narrow borders, where the flowers may be gathered and admired without walking in among them; the taller plants, like columbines, phloxes, and larkspur, behind, and low-growing plants in front. It is the custom to sow annuals in front or between these, but, if space can be afforded, the annuals do much better sown by themselves. For an edging for these narrow beds there is nothing better than box, kept low by shearing every other year. Many people have these borders of hardy flowers in connection with the vegetable garden. Some four feet from the garden wall may be a row of currants, gooseberries, raspberries, swamp peas, or other low-growing bush or tree, and the space between is the hardy flower-garden.

Specialties in the way of flowers are often indulged in. For instance, one may have beds in which in the fall are planted tulips, hyacinths, crocus, or other hardy Dutch bulbs; at the same time lily bulbs may be planted with them. In the spring the Dutch bulbs will fade, and may be carefully taken and planted in some temporary place thickly, to mature. The space between the lilies may then be filled by gladiolus. In this way the one bed has flowers the whole year: hyacinths in spring, lilies in summer, gladiolus in the fall. A good autumn specialty is a collection of plants of the aster and golden-rod family; but separate beds for these imply nothing in bloom for the whole spring and summer. These are better when grown in connection with flowering shrubs, and especially with the rhododendron. Beds of rhododendrons are gaining in popularity from year to year. The soil for them has to be made so light that it will never get dry, and yet have cool, moist air always circulating through it. A well-drained soil, and then filled to a third of its bulk with broken stone, is one of the best rhododendron carpets. These flower in summer. Then around the bed may be a space wide enough for asters, golden-rods, or any plant that flowers freely in the fall. Flowering shrubs give a great attraction to the garden. These are usually scattered over the lawn, or perhaps set in groups here and there on the grass; but excellent effects may often be had by having them occasionally in open beds, and set rather wide, so that the taller and stronger-growing herbaceous plant may be set in front and between. Flowering shrubs, as a rule, have only a week or two for each kind of flower. By a judicious selection something will be in bloom the whole season through; still, there will be many bushes for months without anything, and therefore the introduction of hardy herbaceous plants among them, where it can be done, is an excellent practice.

The rose, of course, is always a favorite specialty, and these are much the best in beds by themselves. A set collection of a number of beds is called a rosery. Whatever design is adopted, the separate beds should always be narrow, so that there shall be no necessity to get in among them. Grass walks kept neatly mown are best for rose-gardens, and not so hot as those of stone or gravel. Those who take great pride in their rose-gardens have trellises and arches in porticos, according to the dictates of taste, on which the climbing varieties are trained.

Trees are not often planted for the flowers they produce so much as for the beauty of their forms or grateful shade. But magnolias, catalpas, paulownias, and some others have many floral attractions besides the pleasure they afford in other respects. In older works of the kind that we are preparing for the reader, it was the custom to give lists of varieties of trees, shrubs, and flowers the cultivator might plant. But the varieties have become so numerous that a book with fresh lists to-day becomes quite stale to-morrow, and, besides, in these days the descriptive catalogues of leading florists and nurserymen are everywhere obtainable by mail. Selections can easily be made, and fresh from year to year. In a general way it may be observed that the chief failure in the cultivation of out-door flowers comes from the poverty of the soil. Flowers want good feeding as well as fruits and vegetables. The soil in the flower-beds should be either frequently changed, which is the best practice, or good well-decayed manure added from year to year.

The leading object in this chapter on gardening has not been to teach the art,—that will have to be studied from more elaborate works,—but rather to occupy a hitherto untrodden field,—the offering of practical suggestions whereby householders may successfully surround themselves by blooming plants all the year round.

SANITARY INFLUENCES OF FOREST-GROWTH.

CHAPTER IX.

Devastation of primitive forests—Evil results from—Conservative influence of forests on the moisture of the soil—Forests feed streams and springs—Relation of forest-growth to malaria—Effects of Eucalyptus plantations upon malaria—Vegetable mould, its advantages and disadvantages—Chemico-vital action of woods—Their mechanical influence to prevent malaria—Forests as preventives of cholera—Their climatic effects—The protective influence of trees by opposing wind-currents—Happy influence of the woodland upon extremes of temperature—The forest air cooler in summer than the open air—Effects of the delicious coolness of shade—Action of woods on the temperature of the air in winter—Their influence upon the humidity of the air—Chiefly due to transpiration—Experiments related—Forest moisture more uniform than that from other sources—Its effects in impeding radiation at night—Experiments by Tyndall—Effects of woods upon the rainfall—Forests as natural ozone-producers—Coniferæ develop ozone actively—Object of wild-flowers in nature—Climatic effects of forests local in character.

THE swiftness with which public as well as professional interest in the subject of forestry has in recent times been increasing may be stated as showing the present to be a peculiarly opportune season for making a calm and exhaustive study of the theme. The subject of the diverse relations of forest-growth to states of climate and the soil embraces numerous important elements, some of which are not only complicating but also really conflicting, and hence has arisen considerable division of opinion among the foremost authorities. Since the higher branches of this science involve issues of leading importance to the public weal, there is no ground for apprehending that the sanitarian will consecrate thereto more investigation than their importance deserves. As every one knows, there was a period in the history of different nations when forests were opined to be practically without limit. As in times coeval with the days of the ancient Greeks and Romans, when "a man was famous according as he *had* lifted up axes upon the thick trees," so already from unknown antiquity our ancestors were celebrated for their industry in felling our own wellnigh limitless timber-growth. The public press as well as scientific writers frequently have been and still are raising a timely cry of warning against the wanton devastation of forest-trees. That such remonstrances are not needless will become clear to any one who will carefully examine the recorded painful experiences of many Oriental countries which have been the result of human improvidence, the physical history of this portion of the globe furnishing numerous and important examples. Of the latter a few striking localities may be mentioned,—namely, Spain, Southern Italy, Persia, Greece, Turkey, and Southern Africa. At a more recent period desolation to an equal degree came upon the French empire, with unequalled suddenness. In England, centuries ago, the rapid disforesting of the woodlands began to excite trepidation for the evil consequences resulting from this course. Owing to the fact that in Germany, France, England, and America very general and lively interest was at an early period excited by this wasteful clearing of the woodland, measures of public policy have been and still are advocated looking to a system of wise management of the forests or the efficient repression of their devastation.

Thus far the almost universal experience of tourists has been that wherever in past time the forests have been cleared away by a populace the effect has been most lamentable, the smaller streams drying up, followed by infertility of soil, insalubrity of climate, and sometimes utter desolation. Frequently associated with the extermination of the forests the population has been observed to be meagre. Though of a negative sort, the above statements evidencing the baneful results of wholesale denudation of the land serve in themselves to indicate the undoubted economic, industrial, and hygienic value of forest-trees to a people. And while it would be an easy task to multiply similar instances indefinitely, from the writings of the best minds of all past ages, to pursue further this line of evidence would be unnecessary, in view of the fact that the writer purposes to bring forward the positive proof at hand, showing how forests favorably affect conditions of soil and climate.

The relation of forest vegetation to the soil and running streams is a subject which has secured the attention of civilized nations of all ages, and it admits of approximate precision of statement; but since it in an indirect way only affects the question of their better climate-influences, its discussion will here be limited to a few general considerations. A leading effect of wooded districts is to preserve the moisture of the soil without favoring excessive humidity of the superficial strata. To account for this it is necessary to consider, first, the action of woods in impeding evaporation from their soil. That savant, Ebermayer, has, as the result of trustworthy meteorological observations on forestry, arrived at the following conclusion: "If from the soil of an open space one hundred parts of water evaporate, then from the soil of a forest free from underwood thirty-eight parts would evaporate, and from a soil covered with underwood only fifteen parts would evaporate." In general, the trees are always supplied with an abundance of moisture for transpiration, owing in great part to the power which the roots have to attract moisture from every direction and to direct the rainfall along their surfaces to great depths, partly to their power of retaining the rainfall in their net-work of smaller rootlets, to be in due season absorbed by the myriads of root-hairs, and partly also to the efficacy of the vegetable mould usually carpeting the soil of the forest to soak up water and prevent its running off rapidly through superficial channels. The action of forests in this regard, it will appear obvious to the reader, must vary greatly in accordance with their situation, being favored more by level than by sloping surfaces. On steep elevations, their effect to nullify destructive avalanches is fully appreciated. The above facts furnish a simple interpretation of how tracts of woodland prevent freshets, which are known to produce marked destructive changes, more especially on the hill-sides and mountainous slopes of unwooded districts. But they are worthy of elaborate mention chiefly as affecting agriculture and other industries of civilized life.

The above facts also explain clearly how forests feed springs and maintain smaller streams on the one hand, and with equal certainty why the clearing of wooded regions causes as a necessary result the drying up of wells, springs, and rivulets.

To show even more conclusively that streams and rivulets owe their origin and permanence to the woodland, they have reappeared after reforesting the places which had been cleared. Again, obviously, this influence of woods is of great importance to the inhabitants of cities, on account of its influence in maintaining and regulating the water-supply. Another evil resulting from the disforesting of a large area is the occurrence of severe droughts, which are quite usually the consequence of excessive surface-drainage, it having been established that less than one-third of the rainfall should directly drain off into the streams. As a matter of practical experience, the people of such localities suffer from frequent floods followed by drought, while their streams are subject to great vacillations. Since the forest soil is at all times provided with an adequate supply for transpiration, not excepting the dry season, and its moisture is ample to keep up the flow of springs perpetually, the equable humidity of forest soil as a factor in obviating droughts, with their baneful consequences to crops of all sorts, with depopulation as the final result, is, in point of practical import, rarely equalled. The fact that the humidity of the forest soil is less variable than that outside sustains important etiological relations to certain epidemic diseases. As has been shown in a previous chapter, the malarial germ, among other essential conditions, demands for its multiplication and development a certain degree of humidity of the soil. The reader should not fail to recount here the remaining concomitants of essential importance to produce the paroxysmal fevers, namely, a temperature not below 67° Fahr. and the direct action of the free oxygen of the air upon the malarial soil. This theory, advanced by Professor Tommasi Crudeli, as before stated, furnishes a satisfactory explanation of numerous phenomena connected with the various expressions of this disorder, hitherto inexplicable. The vexed question, what is the real relationship existing between forest vegetation and soil on the one hand and malarial fevers on the other, has in the past been much, though variously, discussed. The branch of this theme relating to the part played by growing vegetation involves issues which may, for convenience of arrangement, be discussed under three heads: The chemico-vital influence of trees; their mechanical influence in arresting the convection of malaria; their influence upon the humidity of the soil.

With regard to the last element, it is necessary only to state that the physiological functions of vegetable life, transpiration in particular, under ordinary circumstances, tends rather to lessen than to augment the moisture of the forest soil. The foundation of experimental proof, which seems to be ample to establish this proposition, will be hereafter furnished when treating of transpiration from the forest. On the other hand, the value of subsoil drainage, it may be stated, with the view of ridding highly-malarial soil of its redundant moisture, can be proved by a concensus of medical opinion; and in consequence of a full appreciation of this fact, numerous hydraulic systems have been devised, with varying, though on the whole excellent, results. To achieve the same happy object, it has been recommended to plant trees, the number to be proportionate to the needs and extent of any special locality. This application of a scientific principle is best adapted to soils having no natural subsoil drainage, as, for example, in marshy districts, under which conditions they have a decided drying effect. The rate of the process of transpiration, it will be remembered, is practically uniform during clear weather, thus speedily getting rid of the redundancy, especially during dry periods. Again, the trunks of the trees and their branches act as large and efficient reservoirs for the storage of a considerable part of the rainfall; and this is drunk up by the roots almost as soon as precipitated. From these considerations it would naturally be inferred, therefore, that low, marshy ground would be rendered drier by the cultivation of trees in due proportion. Happily, there is historical basis for familiar observations of a practical kind to bear out this idea, though space fails me to cite more than two authorities. In a parliamentary report on the resources and needs of Ireland for forest cultivation, Mr. D. Horwitz, forest conservator of Denmark, observes that "swamps and morasses are created in Ireland from the want of trees to drink up the superfluous moisture." According to the observations of Gimlet, in Algeria, extremely malarious districts have been rendered quite harmless in four or five years by the absorbent action of, and the evaporation from, the leaves of the Eucalyptus globulus. ("Sanitary Influences of Forests," *loc. cit.*, by the author.) Whether or not it is intended to be regarded as a mark of positive superior merit, the writer is not in a position to state, but certain it is that no other species has been placed before the Eucalyptus for drawing moisture from the earth. Physiologically, it is to be remembered that Eucalyptus is an active transpirer, exceeding most other forest species, and its strong aroma must possess correlative powers of purification of the atmosphere; but these seeming advantages are perhaps wholly counterbalanced by the well-known difficulties attending previous efforts at their cultivation in many conditions of climate and soil. And although successfully cultivated in certain malarious localities, they do not invariably furnish immunity from its ravages, since, as pointed out by Professor Tommasi Crudeli, even in the southern hemisphere, the original home of the Eucalyptus, there are Eucalyptus forests which are very malarious; a fact demonstrated by Mr. Liversige, professor in the University of Australia. "Among us also," he continues, "although everybody was convinced by the statements of the press that the locality of the Tre Fontane, near Rome, had been freed from malaria by means of the Eucalyptus, people were disagreeably surprised by an outbreak of very grave fever occurring throughout the whole colony in 1882, a year in which all the rest of the Roman Campagna enjoyed an exceptional salubrity." But to show that this illustrious savant has formed an opinion to some extent in harmony with the view of those observers who have had brought to their observation convincing practical proof of the efficacy of trees in rendering areas of humid soil more wholesome, the following statement, which occurs in the same article, may be quoted: "There is nothing to oppose the admission that these plantations, when properly made, may sometimes have been of great utility." Though it may with confidence be insisted that the balance of testimony is on the side of their beneficial influence in lessening the danger from the damaging activity of the malarial germ, since they strike only at one of the three conditions essential to its development, to go so far as to claim that forests are, under the conditions above outlined, an infallible means of preventing the disease in question, would be to occupy extreme ground. As forests during the cold season distil into the atmosphere little or no moisture, and as their deeper underlying root-terminals, as before explained, after a sponge-like fashion hold considerable moisture in the soil, the earth in their vicinity must be more humid than elsewhere, and it would appear from such considerations that they must prove to be powerful in favoring the development of the specific ferment in the soil in winter; but as one of the requisite conditions is a temperature not below 67° Fahr., malaria, despite the greater humidity of the soil, is rarely developed in winter. It is well to note here that the temperature of the soil which is not exposed to irradiation is 4° C. lower than that of the external soil, that so there may be, and doubtless are, times when the difference between these two localities is of such a degree as that the lower temperature of the forest soil—the latter falling below the required minimum—shall prohibit the production of malaria within the forest, while external to the latter, owing to the higher temperature of the soil there, the malarial ferment may be in process of development and multiplication.

On the other hand, the disease not unfrequently has been observed to prevail extensively in districts where soil contained far less than the average per centum of ground-water. Indeed, whatever differences of opinion may exist as to the conditions to be exacted to produce malaria, it is a remarkable fact that after a heavy rainfall a sinking of the ground-water below a certain level, as, for instance, during a dry period following in the wake of a heavy freshet, malarial outbreaks are both frequent and severe. In explanation of this fact, it may be stated that when the ground-water rises to a high mark the specific ferment may be carried near the exposed surface of the soil, in which situation it would afford opportunity to be operated upon by the two conditions, temperature and the free oxygen of the air, after the subsidence of the ground-water. Having shown forests to be preservers of a uniform degree of moisture in their soil, there can be no gainsaying their effectiveness in securing more or less freedom from malarial infection, under the conditions last named.

Here dawns a remarkable truth: in all unwooded regions where the earth may be wholly dry one day and in consequence of storm subject to flood on the next, forest cultivation would constitute a prompt and efficient means of checkmating not only denudation and threatening unproductiveness of the soil, but also give a greater freedom from insurrections of "shakers." It is an all-important double fact to which earnest attention is here directed, to wit: that in low, moist, or marshy localities forest-culture under proper regulation forms an important factor in lessening the liability to malaria by lessening the humidity of the soil, while in hilly or mountainous regions forest-growth likewise lessens the liability to this affection by maintaining a more rigidly uniform standard of moisture than outside, though in different degrees. The present inquiry, it should be noted, does not refer to residence under the shadow of an extended area of woods, but to a habitat in proximity to the latter, if regard be paid to the needs of the locality and to geographical distribution, the rules for which will be pointed out hereafter. The writer is fully aware that treatises by eminent writers upon the same subject frequently take a different view, contending that forests have a twofold effect,—namely, that of greatly increasing the humidity of the soil and contributing with equal certainty to render the climate insalubrious, more especially favoring the prevalence of malarial diseases. Nor can this opinion be said to be leagued with fanaticism, since universal experience has proved it to be sound under certain conditions of topography and character of forest species. If, for instance, reference be had only to the deep, dense forests of the tropical regions, with their luxuriant undergrowth of humble vegetation and their thick covering of vegetable mould in a partial state of decay, there is truth in the proposition that plantations moisten the soil to an extent undesirable, and tend to augment the danger from malaria to an equal degree. But we are here contending for the beneficial effects of forests under widely different conditions, or, in other words, for the favorable influence of woods *in fair proportion in temperate climates* under the direction of competent authority. The forests of old, above alluded to, are objectionable because of their greater density and because they embrace enormous areas of territory, though in still greater part owing to the presence of thick bibulous humus overlying the soil of the forest, which latter condition forms an excellent receptacle for the malarial germ in districts naturally malarious, being sufficiently moist, thus placing it in conditions most favorable to be acted upon by the warm climate and the free oxygen of the atmosphere. This observation, though true of the extensive tropical forests, is wholly inapplicable to the presence of a per centum of woodland such as necessary for climatic influences in temperate climates, so that the justice of our position is not disproved by it. The consideration of the sanitary effects of the humus overlying the forest soil is here arrived at, and deserves a moment's attention. It presents difficulties of considerable magnitude. Humus, as before incidentally pointed out, has some advantages, and equal certain disadvantages. The benefits of vegetable mould from a sanitary point of view should be restated. They are: the power it possesses to absorb a portion of the rainfall and prevent it coursing down hills and mountain-slopes, causing superficial erosions, and for a like reason to assist to preserve the moisture in the soil of the forest. It is also an active agency in promoting the fertility of the forest soil. A positively disappointing influence of humus, if it be very thick, is to produce an increased dampness of the superficial strata in all places, save when located on the steeper slopes. In this humid state of the surface-soil and of the heavy layer of humus covering it, lies, for reasons above given, an imminent danger of bringing about those concauses which result in the production of malaria. A practical lesson may be drawn from this simple fact; that is, the importance of thinning out the dense underbrush and removing the injurious covering of mould, in regions known to be malarial. This could be accomplished without cause for being apprehensive of the evil consequences in the way of physical deterioration, and such a course would also facilitate evaporation from the soil, while the moisture not evaporated would, as is always the case, be conveyed by the roots to the deeper strata far beyond the reach of surface-evaporation. For obvious reasons, such a precaution is to be deemed unnecessary on precipitous mountain-slopes. To allow more than a meagre proportion of mould and underbrush in general is a matter of the utmost importance, demanding that it should form the basis of a suitable public policy. In concluding the present discussion of the relation of forest-growth to humidity of soil and the origin and the dispersion of the malarial diseases, it remains to be pointed out that the greater equanimity of the moisture of the forest soil is in some measure to be accounted for by the fact that the rainfall is more evenly distributed than in unwooded districts. Notwithstanding the fact that forests effect a conservation of the moisture of the soil, there are, it should be remarked, numerous wooded districts, even on high elevations, under the shadows of whose forests malarial diseases rarely or never occur.

The chemico-vital action of forests in counteracting

malarial diseases is an aspect of the subject which may be disposed of summarily, since this may be said to be but slight. Of all the attainable facts pertaining thereto, none afford satisfactory evidence that their physiological processes, or any emanations resulting from the latter, exercise the desirable effect of being in any sense antidotal to this ferment, except the function of the generation of ozone, which, though it cannot destroy by oxidation the disease-producing germs, must, however, destroy much of the organic atmospheric impurities acting as disease-carriers. Owing to the strong absorbing powers of forest-growth and humble vegetation generally, a purifying influence of no mean importance is exercised upon the soil, which is frequently more or less befouled by the products of surface-drainage from the nearest habitations. Upon this point Professor von Pettenkofer pertinently remarks: "If this refuse matter remains in soil destitute of growing vegetation, further decomposition sets in, and other processes are induced not always of a salubrious nature, but often deleterious, the products of which reach us by means of air or water, and many penetrate into our house." Although living vegetation sucks up much of the waste products which must be regarded as hurtful, and would otherwise be returned in the form of vapor to the superjacent atmosphere, there is no positive proof of the fact that the malarial germ can be thus rendered innocuous; or, in other words, that growing vegetable life, owing to its strong powers of imbibition from the soil, is to be regarded as a prophylactic measure against the disease under discussion.

SANITARY INFLUENCES OF FOREST-GROWTH. 271

As has been frequently remarked by writers on the subject, trees in belts or masses, or even heavy shrubbery placed between the originating places of the germs of malaria and human habitations, afford efficient protection from paroxysmal diseases. From the wonderful unanimity of recorded observations by physicians living in malarial districts, this fact may be looked upon as proved beyond peradventure.

How is the effect in question produced? High authority, Professors Flint and Metcalfe among others, believes that the malarial germ has a peculiar affinity for vegetable life as well as organic matter in general.

Though thought by most authorities to be effected mechanically, this observation and the underlying principle it involves have up to within a recent period been regarded as really inexplicable;-but there is afforded a probable interpretation by the results of some simple experiments by Professor Tyndall.

He found that the air of enclosed boxes at the expiration of three days no longer contained any of the microscopical particles invariably suspended in ordinary air, these having all attached themselves to the sides of the boxes. Into similar boxes he introduced different infusions of meat and vegetables, which for weeks and months remained unchanged, while, as was to be expected, when the same infusions were exposed to the general atmosphere, they speedily underwent decomposition, becoming alive with bacteria. ("Floating Matter in the Air," John Tyndall, F.R.S., 1882; quoted by J. F. A. Adams, "Sanitary Forest-culture," 1884.) If, then, minute air-borne matter has an affinity for organic surfaces indifferently, it can be easily seen how vegetable growth, by arresting the onward passage of atmospheric currents, would attract to itself mites carrying the malarial germ. These simple experiments appear to demonstrate the mode of bringing about this happy issue, this being purely mechanical. Since the ability on the part of vegetable forms, be they large or small, to intercept the specific cause of malaria is not confined to those species which develop ozone, there can be no basis for the theory that the ozone generated by plant life is the exclusive agent in nullifying the effects of this specific ferment.

To present numerous illustrations of the influence of forests in question, as, for instance, examples in which the removal of trees suitably located to protect against malaria was followed by an outbreak of the disease, would not prove to be a difficult task; but as this has been frequently done by medical writers we need to adduce but two, which are quite typical. Though oft quoted as an evidence of the practicability of trees as efficient intercepters, the clearing away of the forest-growth between the Pontine marshes and the city of Rome more than a century ago, at the request of Pope Benedict against the recalcitrations of Lancisci, should be placed foremost.

The result in this instance was a decided outbreak of malaria in Rome, in some portions of which it was so virulent as to render them uninhabitable.

A few rows of sunflowers, planted between the Washington Observatory and the marshy banks of the Potomac, in the opinion of Lieutenant Maury, had defended the inmates of that establishment from the paroxysmal fevers to which they were formerly liable. In Italy

Maury's experiments have been repeated. Large plantations of sunflowers have been made upon the alluvial deposits of Oglio, above its entrance into the Lake of Isco, near Pisogne, and it is said with favorable results to the health of the neighborhood (Marsh, G. P., "Man and Nature," *loc. cit.*, pp. 154, 155; quoted from Saloagnoli, *Memoirii Sulle*, Maremme Iascani, pp. 213, 214).

In later times the observation has been repeatedly made by competent authorities that variations in the moisture of the soil, to the extent either of rising above or falling below a certain level, exerts a marked influence upon the prevalence and fatality of typhoid fever and cholera; while conversely, if the degree of humidity remains within certain limits of variation, these diseases are not so likely to become epidemic. Applying the facts before adduced in regard to the action of forests upon the moisture in the soil, their obvious effect to lessen the prevalence of the diseases last mentioned requires no commentary.

Practically, Von Pettenkofer, who is the most earnest champion of this school, has shown how forests and plantations act as efficient preventives of cholera. " It has always been observed," he tells us, " that villages in wooded districts suffer less from the disease than those in treeless plains." He proceeds: " Many instances of this are given in the reports of Dr. Bryden (president of the Statistical Office in Calcutta) and Dr. Murray, inspector of hospitals. For instance, Bryden ("Epidemic Cholera in the Bengal Presidency," 1869, p. 225) compares the district of the Mahanadda, one of the northern tributaries of the Ganges, the almost treeless district of the Rajpoor, with the district of Sambalpoor. It is stated that in the villages in the plain of Rajpoor sixty or seventy per cent. of the inhabitants are sometimes swept away by cholera in three or four days, while the wooded district of Sambalpoor is often free from it, or it is much less severe. The district commissioner, who had to make a tour in the district on account of the occurrence of cholera, reports among other things as follows: "The road to Sambalpoor runs for sixty or seventy miles through the forest, which around Petorah and Jenkfluss is very dense. Now it is a remarkable fact, but it is a fact nevertheless, that on this route, traversed daily by hundreds of travellers, vehicles, and baggage-trains, the cholera rarely appears in this extent of sixty miles, and when it does appear it is in a mild form; but when we come from the road from Arang, westward to Chicholee Bungalow, which runs for about ninety miles through a barren, treeless plain, we find the cholera every year in its more severe form, the dead and dying lying by the wayside, and trains of vehicles half of whose conductors are dead." A striking instance showing the influence of trees on the spread of cholera is given by Murray (quoted by Von Pettenkofer) as follows: "The fact is generally believed, and not long ago the medical officer of Jatisgas, in Central India, offered a striking proof of it. During the widespread epidemic of cholera in Allahabad, in 1859, those parts of the garrison whose barracks had the advantage of having trees near them enjoyed an indisputable exemption, and precisely in proportion to the thickness and nearness of the shelter. Thus the European Cavalry in the Wellington Barracks, which stand between four rows of mango-trees, but are yet to a certain extent open, suffered much less than the Fourth European Regiment, whose quarters were on a hill exposed to the full force of the wind; while the Bengal Horse Artillery, who were in a picket of mango-trees, had not a single case of sickness; and the exemption cannot be regarded as accidental, as the next year the comparative immunity was precisely the same." ("Report on the Treatment of Epidemic Cholera," 1869, p. 4.)

In his paper Von Pettenkofer proceeds: "We need not, however, go to India to observe similar instances of the influence of a certain degree of moisture in the soil favored by woods or other conditions; we can find them much nearer home. In the cholera epidemic of 1854, in Bavaria, it was generally observed that the places in the moors were spared, in spite of the otherwise bad condition of the inhabitants. The great plain of the Danube, from Neuburg to Ingolstadt, was surrounded by places where it was epidemic, while in the plain itself there were but a few scattered cases. The same thing has been demonstrated by Reinhard, president of the Saxon Medical College. Cholera has visited Saxony eight times since 1836, and every time it spared the northerly district between Pleisse and Spree, where ague is endemic.

"In the English Garden at Munich there are several buildings not sparsely tenanted,—the Diana Baths, the Chinese Tower, with a tavern and out-buildings, the Gendarmerie Station, and the Kleinkessellohe. In the three outbreaks of cholera at Munich, none of these places have been affected by it. This fact is the more surprising, as three of them comprise public taverns, into which the disease-germs must have been occasionally introduced by the public; yet there was no epidemic in these houses, although it prevailed largely immediately beyond the English Garden and close to the Diana Baths in 1854 and 1873. It must have been accidental that no isolated cases occurred, as the inmates of the Chinese Tower or the Kleinkessellohe might have caught it in Munich, as others did who came from a distance; but had there been single cases probably no epidemic would have occurred in these houses. Even if these deductions must be accepted with caution from an etiological point of view, still, on the whole, they indisputably tell in favor of trees and woods."

Of all the effects of forest-growth, the purely climatic are to be regarded as being of greatest philosophical interest and practical significance, though they undeniably involve inquiries which are both difficult and obscure. About the year 1864, Marsh (*loc. cit.*, p. 194), in discussing the meteorological influence of forests, remarked that the conclusions of physicists respecting them are in a great degree inferential, only not founded on experiment or direct observation. Under such circumstances it will not be surprising to the reader who has not already informed himself upon this particular issue to learn that prior to the above period the conclusions reached by leading authorities were quite inharmonious. While space fails me to discuss the various views of the older writers, and which discussion could lead to no useful results, it may aid in interesting the reader to note that the latest and best light thrown upon the main elements of the question has been in the shape of knowledge gained by direct experiment, and therefore of a nature calculated to settle some of the points involved definitely. The balance of argument and opinion to-day (March, 1886), it may be truthfully alleged, is on the side in favor of the marked beneficial climatic effects of forest vegetation. It is but fair to observe, however, that a few observers of note deny any effects of woods upon the leading climatic elements, namely, temperature, humidity, and so on; but this assumption rests, we think, on too slender evidence to be entitled to credence. It may with confidence be assumed that forests affect favorably the chief meteorological conditions, if we except special cases, or, in other words, regions where the natural advantages of climate are perhaps unequalled.

One of the ways in which forests exert an influence upon the climate is by opposing resistance to the free passage of wind-currents. This element of the question, though, perhaps, more firmly established than any other, is of too great importance to be disposed of in a summary manner. Evidently trees are well adapted to break the force of the winds, since the branches, and particularly the leaves, on account of their immense numbers and nearness to one another, act as efficient bearers; the trunk in turn, holding up the bushy tree-top, defies the tempest, while the roots on their part are extending their grip on "mother earth" in order to support the stem. The particles of air not checked by the first row of trees to the windward would, it is clear, have their force diminished, and would be promptly checked by the trees to the rear. In this manner considerable masses or even belts of trees, by intercepting strong wind-currents, afford shelter to man, the crops, and humbler vegetation generally to the leeward, from the chilly blasts of winter as well as the drying winds of summer, thus having the effect to modify extremes of temperature, rendering summer less sultry and winter less severe.

In tempering chilly spring and autumn winds, they lengthen relatively the warm season or term of vegetable growth and development. To the agriculturist this fact is highly important, since on the one hand certain crops are slow in maturing, and on the other the bleak winds are in many unwooded regions known to be highly unfavorable to the maturation of fruit-crops and harvests. It has been many times observed that, given similar soils, fruit grown in the city surpasses in quality and size that grown in the country,—a fact ascribable to the more effectual shelter in the former than in the latter locality.

Of little less importance, perhaps, is the effect exercised by forests in protecting from the drying winds of midsummer, which are frequently the cause of blighted crops and of other mischief, producing their untoward results by enhancing evaporation from vegetation and the open soil during the dry season. For similar reasons, there is need of woods ever on our coasts. The sea-breezes on striking the land become warmed, whereby their capacity for moisture is greatly increased, thus naturally absorbing the earth's moisture with avidity and producing a parching influence. In France the experiment of planting trees in belts one hundred metres apart has been tried, and with marked benefit to the climate, and the practice has been thought to be worthy of imitation in our own and other countries.

As has already been incidentally mentioned, the temperature of the soil of the woodland is several degrees lower than that outside. According to Ebermayer, the trunks of the trees "breast-high" are 5° Centigrade lower in temperature than the air of the forest; but this difference of temperature, it is to be noted, is nearly maintained when comparing the temperature of the tops of the forest-trees with the forest air. Ebermayer speaks of the temperature of the trees in a forest as being *always* lower than the air of the forest. This admits of easy explanation: the rapid transpiration of watery vapor from the foliage, beautifully shown by our own researches (*supra*), renders the action of the solar rays neutral, thus reducing the temperature considerably.

During the warm season the air of the forest is cooler than the open air,—a fact due to several co-operative influences. As will be hereafter demonstrated, the air of the forest contains a somewhat higher standard of average humidity, and any increase in the amount of moisture in the air it is well understood reduces the temperature, though the fall is not always proportional. That eminent physician, Dr. Frankland, is made to say that he considers the moisture in the atmosphere of England as lowering the temperature from fifteen to twenty-five degrees (Dr. Blodget, *Journal American Medical Association*, August 23, 1884).

An eminent Russian observer, M. Woeikoff, has recently called attention to the depressing effect of moisture upon the temperature (Peterman's "Mittheilungen," *Pop. Science Mo.*, January, 1886, pp. 428–430). After stating a well-known fact, to wit, the gradual increase in the normal temperature as we go from the sea toward the interior in Western Europe and Asia, he sets forth the power of a forest to compensate for the rise in temperature: "so that there are places far from the sea that are cooler than the shore itself. This is the case in Bosnia, where the summer is five or six degrees cooler than in Herzegovina, on account of the woods."

It is of cardinal importance to note that this action of forests upon the temperature is extended, through the currents, for some distance in every direction. Again, the screen formed by the branches and foliar organs to a great degree intercept the solar rays, causing shade, which has a delightfully cooling effect. As has been pointed out by Von Pettenkofer, shade in the open air always causes a slight draft, "which acts as a kind of fan." This he correctly explains as follows: "So far as the shade extends the air is cooler than in the sun; layers of air of unequal warmth are of different gravity, and this difference of temperature is the cause of the motion in the air." Doubtless, all of our readers have experienced the refreshing coolness of shade on passing from without into a dense grove in excessively warm weather. But let us look a little deeper, and inquire how this peculiarly delightful effect is produced. In a previous chapter the power which the human body possesses to regulate its own temperature was alluded to in speaking of the evil consequences of living in an atmosphere having a changeable temperature and humidity. The normal temperature of the body (98° Fahr.) cannot be exceeded, if we would wish to enjoy good health or to feel comfortable. During the oppressive heat of midsummer the body generates more heat than during the other seasons, or, more correctly stated, the body parts with the excess of heat less readily; the loss by radiation being greatly impeded on account of the high temperature of the surrounding objects and the atmosphere, while the greater evaporation of moisture from the skin must compensate therefor. Now, when we enter a densely-shaded woodland we feel a delicious coolness, partly on account of the moderating influences of the gentle breezes encountered, but chiefly on account of the radiation of heat by contact with a medium of lower temperature.

In many flowers it is well known there is considerable heat developed preceding and during fecundation. The temperature of certain arums has been observed to rise more than 10° Fahr. Though this phenomenon may be universal, it is doubtless subject to great variation, while none, so far as known by botanists, equal the *arum* in the evolution of heat. Reasoning from this analogy, the flowers of the forest-trees, certain writers have contended, must, during the flowering stage, exert an important influence on the warmth of the atmospheric strata in contact with them. But, as will appear evident to the reader, this cannot atone for the various counter-influences which tend to reduce the temperature during the warm season. There is yet another aspect of this branch of our theme worthy of brief consideration, the substance of it being embraced in the following query, namely, How does the temperature of the woodland air compare with the air devoid of vegetable growth in winter? In his valuable work on "Man and Nature" (p. 157), Marsh quotes Megrascher (*Memoria sui Boschi de Lombardia*, p. 45), according to whom observation shows that the trees have a more uniform temperature than the atmosphere, or, in other words, the internal warmth of the trees does not rise and fall proportional to that of the atmosphere in general. He further contends: so long as the temperature of the latter is below 67° Fahr., that of the tree is the higher; but if the temperature of the air rises to 67° Fahr., then the tree marks the lowest. Without stopping to discuss this opinion, which appears to rest upon exact scientific premises, it is to be remarked that, if it be true, it affords another evidence of the cardinal fact that forests are natural equalizers of temperature, since such observations indisputably teach that the air encircling the forest is warmer in winter than the external.

No other influence which forests exert upon climate, however, can claim so large a share of importance as that exercised upon the humidity of the air. The explanation of their effect upon this meteorological element is to be found in a study of the organic process previously discussed, namely, transpiration; but in some slight degree also in their mechanical influence. Among the latter effects there is to be observed, as before noted, the vegetable canopy above, which prevents in a great measure the rays of the sun from reaching the earth and warming it so as to facilitate evaporation from the soil. Again, by forming a more or less perfect screen interposed between sky and earth, forests in a measure intercept the dews and lighter rains, which are at once returned to the atmosphere by evaporation, a small portion of this moisture only reaching the earth. The evaporation from the soil of the forest, computed by Ebermayer, *supra*, is rather more than one-third as great as that from open soil, but this lessened surface-evaporation is much more than counterbalanced by the transpiration from the forest, as will be indicated elsewhere by the results of our investigation.

In approaching the discussion of the effect of the organic functions upon the humidity of the air, we reach a most interesting and vitally-important question. The power possessed by forest-trees to absorb moisture from the deeper strata of the earth is sufficient evidence to show that they are always supplied with enough water to meet the demands of nutrition and transpiration, seeing that the view claiming the green portions and foliar organs of trees as organs of absorption of moisture from the atmosphere under these circumstances, is, as before demonstrated, inadmissible. The only physiological function which, from facts of observation really produces a marked effect upon this meteorological element is, therefore, transpiration, which has already received the attention this highly-attractive subject demands, so far as relates to such leading inquiries as its rate, true nature, and effect upon the extent of saturation of the air in enclosed rooms. However, we shall incidentally draw upon the principles deduced from our previous researches when necessary to make plain points which we shall regard as being germane to the present discussion. Thus, at the outset the reader should not fail to recall the great activity of this function ("Transpiration of Plants," *loc. cit.*), the rate at which aqueous vapor is given off by plants being rather more than one and a quarter ounces per square foot of leaf-surface for twelve diurnal hours. If the reader will reflect for a moment upon the vast expanse of leaf-area of a single tree emitting vapor at this rate; if he will also consider the total number of trees in a forest composed of but a few acres, the number per acre being variously estimated at from one hundred and fifty to six hundred trees, and multiplying these two factors the product will in some degree give an approximate idea of the enormity of the quantity of water which forests supply to our atmosphere in a highly-acceptable form. Surely, forests are great natural dispensers of moisture. From the general statements just adduced, it would seem to me to be entirely warrantable to draw the *a priori* conclusion, namely, that wherever a fair proportion of woodland exists, a considerable influence is thereby exerted upon the hydrometeorology of a region. The accuracy of this proposition, though apparently logically sound, has been set at rest by the writer in a published paper on "Forests—their Influence upon Climate and Rainfall" (*Amer. Nat.*, Jan., 1882, pp. 19–30), from which paper the following citation will be given a place here:

"During the past summer I have instituted a series of experiments with the view of determining the amount vaporized from known areas of leaf-surface, land-surface, and water under similar conditions, in order that an approximately correct estimate of evaporation from these various sources might be made.

"A pot-plant having one square foot of leaf-surface was carefully prepared in the manner described (in a previous chapter), so as to prevent any evaporation from the pot in which it was growing. Another glazed pot was filled with soil (a light clay loam) so as to expose a surface of only twenty-four square inches, the pot being about the same size as that containing the plant, and its depth being very nearly six inches. The plant was sufficiently watered to keep it in a thrifty condition, while the earth in the plantless pot was kept generally well saturated. Both were exposed to the outer air. The evaporation from earth and plant was now tested simultaneously by weighing the two pots at stated intervals, and it was found that the mean evaporation in fair weather was nearly equal for the two sources, with a slight preponderance on the side of the soil. For fourteen consecutive days of clear and partly cloudy weather, the mean transpiration from the plant was a little over one and a quarter ounces, and the evaporation from the soil one and a third ounces. This would place the rate of evaporation of equal areas of leaf and land surface, under like circumstances of exposure, at about six to one in favor of the soil; that is to say, one square foot of soil will evaporate six times as much as one square foot of leaf-surface. This will appear quite plain when it is remembered that the extent of leaf-surface was exactly six times as great as that of the soil, and that the diurnal evaporation was so nearly equal from the two sources. These experiments were several times repeated with similar results.

"Now, if it were known how many times greater the leaf-surface of a forest is than the land on which it is situated, it might with ease be computed what is the relative evaporation from a forest and an equal area of open country. From personal observations we think it safe to assume that the leaf-surface of a wooded district is at least twelve times as great as that of the ground on which it stands, so that at the above rate the transpiration from the forest would be nearly twice as great as the evaporation from an equal area of open soil. It should be mentioned also that the evaporation from the earth in this case was under the most favorable circumstances, and the state of the ground as regards moisture was very like that of the earth directly after a moderate rain. The evaporation from the soil in the pot was found by testing to be nearly equal to that given off by a similar area of water. It would appear certain from these investigations that more water is emitted to the air from a forest than from an equal body of water, and in this there is a confirmation of the experiments of Williams, who computed the evaporation from a wood to be one-third more than an equal space covered with water (Agriculture Report for 1865, p. 526). It is well known that at times, more particularly during the warm season, we have no rain for several weeks together, so that the mean general surface evaporation is probably not by any means as great as would be indicated by these figures; for it was found that by allowing the soil in the pot to become even moderately dry, the amount evaporated would fall far short of what it was when keeping the soil well watered. On the other hand, there are good reasons for believing that the true rate at which forests give out aqueous vapor is at all events not overestimated in these researches, since, as before pointed out, the trees are at all times supplied with an abundance of moisture which they pump up from the deeper strata.

"The humbler specimens of vegetation also have an effect in the same direction, as is conclusively shown by the following experiment: A pot with artificially-prepared soil, similar to that used in the above experiments, was used. Another vessel of the same size and weight, in which grass (*Poa annua*) about four inches high was growing, was simultaneously employed. Now it was found by repeated testing that from the pot containing the grass the evaporation exceeded that of the pot containing only soil. The rates in ounces would be about five to four for the grass and soil, respectively.

"From the data just obtained it would seem safe to infer that when the percentage of woodland is fair, say from twenty-five to thirty per cent., at least twelve inches of water is transpired in the course of a season in a mild or temperate climate, or, in other words, twelve inches of the total annual terrestrial evaporation."

As tending to support the above dictum, the experiments of L. Fantiat and A. Sartiaux (translation of a communication to the French Academy of Sciences, *Pop. Sc. Mo.* for June, 1875) are of great value and not less interesting. From this communication a brief note will be here incorporated. They say, "We now made the following observations in the heart of the forest of Helatt, which embraces five thousand hectares of land. At the height of about six metres (say twenty feet), above a group of oaks and hornbeans eight or nine metres high, we placed a pluviometer, psychrometer, maxima and minima thermometers, and an evaporometer, so as to ascertain at that point the amount of rainfall, the degree of saturation of the air, and the rate of temperature and evaporation. In open air at a distance of only three hundred metres from the forest, and at the same height above the ground, as in the former case, we placed similar instruments under the same conditions. With regard to the rainfall and the degree of saturation, the observations for six months show the total rainfall to be 192.50 mm. in the forest, and 177 mm. in the open air; differences in favor of the forest, 15.50 mm. The degree of humidity for the open air showed a mean of 61.7°, and in the forest 63°, the difference in favor of the forest, 1.3°."

As above shown, transpiration is not governed by the same physical laws as evaporation from soil and water,—a fact of the greatest import, since implying less variation in the amount of moisture exhaled by growing vegetation than in the rate of terrestrial evaporation, thus insuring a more rigidly uniform degree of humidity in the vicinity of sylvan flora. Apart from the evident advantages of forest humidity above alluded to, this phase of our discussion has still another aspect, which we have designated as the indirect effect of transpiration, embracing hygienic principles whose importance stands almost unequalled (see *ante*, chap. v.). As an instance, we may mention the important office on the part of atmospheric moisture in impeding the radiation of the earth's heat.

The term radiation has been defined by Professor Tyndall as a "vibratory movement which begins in the ultimate particles of matter, and is propagated through waves of ether." Bodies which will allow the rays of light to pass freely through them are said to be transparent; on the other hand, bodies allowing radiant heat to pass through them are said to be diathermic. In every body the absorption and radiation of heat are reciprocal. The diathermacy of different substances, it has been found experimentally, is greatly modified by certain conditions, among which may be mentioned the nature of the molecules of the body, its thickness, and especially the source, or, to speak more accurately, the kind of heat. The rays of heat which are not transmissible through a body are absorbed by it, thus elevating its temperature, but when the body is perfectly diathermic there is no elevation of temperature ("Beneficial Influence of Plants," by the author, *loc. cit.*, pp. 801, 802). As the substance with which we at present writing are solely concerned—aqueous vapor in the air—is in the gaseous state, we shall turn our attention to this class of substances. And since some solid and liquid bodies are nearly, and in a few instances wholly, diathermic, to speak of gases absorbing and radiating heat may at first sight strike the reader as being chimerical; and if we reflect upon the greater spaces between the molecules of the latter as compared with the former, the interception of rays by these particles seems truly monstrous. But the skilful and delicate experimentation by Professor Tyndall has placed beyond the pale of mere reasoning the fact that gases also absorb and radiate heat, though this is not the place to describe the methods pursued and the apparatus used by this noted investigator. It must suffice to note a few of his conclusions. It seems to be due to Professor Tyndall to remark our utmost confidence in the accuracy of the results he obtained, after a perusal of his admirable work on "Radiation," where everything is fully explained. Among some of the commoner vapors and gases he found extreme variations as to their absorbent powers. Thus on the one hand the capacity of hydrogen and of dry air to absorb radiant heat were found to be inconspicuously small, while on the other carbon monoxide and carbon dioxide were shown to be active absorbents. Considering the absorbing capacity of dry air to be one, that of carbon dioxide would be ninety. Experiments with ozone placed this substance in the foremost ranks as an intercepter of radiant caloric. Though perhaps not strictly pertinent to the subject, the conclusions cited are certainly of great scientific interest and importance. Happily for our purpose, this illustrious scientist has not omitted to study the effect on radiant heat of the watery vapor constantly present in our atmosphere. The following observations relative to this constituent of the atmosphere from the author's own writings (*loc. cit.*, pp. 804, 805) should here be incorporated: "The quantity of vapor of water contained in the air is very small indeed, constituting only about four and a half per cent., and although the moisture is everywhere present, its ratio is very variable. It is perfectly invisible, so that by our senses we are quite unable to judge of the amount present; even the purest sky may contain a large proportion. As this vapor is to all intents and purposes a gaseous body, obeying the laws of gases, any one not familiar with the information we have just outlined would doubtless hesitate to accept the assertion that the watery vapor so sparsely scattered through the atmosphere is the main agent in regulating the nocturnal radiation from the earth's surface. Even Professor Tyndall himself for some time neglected this substance; and, in his own phraseology, could hardly credit the first results which made the action of the aqueous vapor of the laboratory fifteen times that of the air in which it was diffused. But this result does not show the correct relation of the action of vapor and air, for after repeated experiments with air from different localities, and examined similarly, the results were uniformly to the effect that vapor of water has an absorbing capacity seventy times that of the air in which it is contained. Many objections and criticisms, some of which seemed almost unsurmountable, were overcome by varying the methods of procedure. The assertion above made seems to have been fully and satisfactorily demonstrated by a most careful and competent experimentalist.

"Still further testimony might be adduced, the result of observations by meteorologists.

"Colonel Richard Strache, an eminent meteorologist, made observations showing the relation between the tension of the aqueous vapor of the atmosphere and the fall of the thermometer during the night. A single statement taken from his results will be ample for our purpose, namely, When the tension of vapor was 0.888 inches the fall of the thermometer was 6° Fahr., and when the tension was only 0.435 inches the fall amounted to 16.5° Fahr. It is just to state that these observations were conducted long before Professor Tyndall's researches with aqueous vapor, and are on this account all the more valuable."

The evidence we have adduced seems to show conclusively that the vapor in the air forms a sort of invisible canopy separating the chilling air above from the warm earth beneath, and arresting more or less effectually the radiation. We have a homely illustration of this when we see the thrifty housewife spread coverings over the more delicate plants of her flower-garden on nights when she fears frost.

It has been said that the aqueous vapor in the air is a blanket more necessary to the vegetable life of England than clothing is to man; and every plant capable of destruction by freezing would succumb if this were removed for a single night. In support of this assertion, it is well to notice the results attained by a few noted observers concerning daily fluctuations in the temperature in different countries. Dr. Livingstone has observed a great excess in nocturnal chilling when the air is dry over that which occurred when it is laden with moisture. He has found in the southern and central portions of Africa, during the month of June, the thermometer early in the morning at from 42° to 50° Fahr., at noon 94° to 96° Fahr., or a mean difference of 48° Fahr. between sunrise and mid-day. He says, further, "The sensation of cold after the heat of the day was very keen. The Bolanda at this season never make their fires until nine or ten in the morning. As the cold was so great here, it was probably frosty at Liganti; I therefore feared to expose very young trees there."

("Livingstone's Travels," p. 484.) Crossing the continent, Dr. Livingstone reaches the Zambezi at the commencement of the year. He gives the following description of the river: "We were struck by the fact that as soon as we came between the range of the hills which flanked the Zambezi the rains felt warm. At sunrise the thermometer stood at from 82° to 86° Fahr.; at mid-day, in the coolest shade in the middle of my little tent under a shady tree, at 96° to 98° Fahr., and at sunset at 86° Fahr. This is different from anything we experienced in the interior" (*loc. cit.*, p. 575). . . .

In Australia the daily range of temperature is extremely great. The observations of Mr. W. S. Jevons (quoted by Tyndall) are of much interest, and hence we give an extract: "In the interior of the continent of Australia the fluctuations in temperature are immensely increased. The heat of the air, as described by Captain Stewart, is fearful during summer; thus, in about latitude 30° 50'', and longitude 141° 18' E., he writes: 'The thermometer every day rose to 112° or 116° in the shade, while in the direct rays of the sun from 140° to 150°. Again, at quarter-past 3 P. M., on June 21, 1845, the thermometer had risen to 131° in the shade, 154° in the direct rays of the sun. . . . In the winter the thermometer was observed as low as 24°, giving an extreme range of 107°.'"

Says Professor Tyndall: "Without quitting Europe, we find places where, while the day temperature is very high, an hour before sunrise is very cold. I have often experienced this in the post wagons of Germany; and I am informed that the Hungarian peasants, if exposed at night, take care, even in hot weather, to protect themselves by heavy cloaks against the nocturnal chill."

All this evidence should be sufficient to convince the most sceptical that the aqueous vapor of the air furnishes a quite efficient barrier to terrestrial radiation. As all know, nature's chief means of furnishing this essentially-important substance is through evaporation from the ocean, especially in the tropics, but many inland regions, and even certain tracts near the great seas, do not, owing to forest denudation and other causes, contain the needful extent of moisture in the air.

If the writer has been successful in showing that a large proportion of the atmospheric moisture may be accounted for through the process of transpiration,—that is, where a fair per centum of woodland is afforded by a region of country,—and if a proportional degree of humidity exerts an important influence upon the daily temperature range and other meteorological questions, then the public significance of the practice of sylviculture in districts not properly wooded cannot be too strongly emphasized.

A low humidity, our readers will now perceive, admits of active radiation, and in consequence great nocturnal fall and daily variation in temperature, which latter conditions prevail at high altitudes, and, as heretofore pointed out, form the main objection to these climes. And here is another extremely significant fact,—namely, forests distil their moisture into the atmosphere with greater uniformity of rate than

SANITARY INFLUENCES OF FOREST-GROWTH. 295

occurs from other surfaces, the soil or water, for example, thus, happily, giving us a more equable climate, with smaller fluctuations in temperature, which conditions, as before intimated, so far as pertains to public health, are of higher importance than the average temperature of the seasons.

From the results of our experimental labors the reader will remember it was shown that the presence of forest-growth to the extent of one-fourth the total acreage may account for the equivalent of twelve inches of the rainfall during the annual period of vegetable growth, by the phenomenon of transpiration; and, in view of this demonstrated truth, the reader is pardonable for thinking it a natural corollary that timberland has the power of increasing the annual rainfall. But the old question, Do forests in any degree influence the rainfall? is not as yet quite satisfactorily determined, since the total annual evaporation and precipitation bear a constant relation. That they do not, therefore, augment the total rainfall may be regarded as a thing definitely settled. But, on the other hand, the woodland does possess a local influence upon precipitation, promoting gentle showers, and, within certain areas of space and limits of time, influence both the amount and distribution. Their influence in these tendencies can be well understood by attention to the nature of certain meteorological phenomena. The question where and in what manner is the moisture given to the air by a forest condensed into rain needs to be answered here. It is well first to note that rain, according to well-known meteorological principles, is usually formed at great heights, say from one to two miles above the earth's surface, hence it cannot reasonably be claimed that woods under ordinary circumstances materially affect the general course of storms. Forest-growth when situated on mountains, besides favoring in a mechanical manner the ascent of vapor-laden currents to cooler regions where condensation occurs, might also, owing to their altitude, have their own moisture condensed into rain. Situated upon a level tract or upon low elevations, the conditions are vastly less favorable. However, if the reader will reflect upon the demonstrable variations in the temperature of the air of forests and the currents outside, as before fully explained, and the circumstance of these atmospheres commingling, it will doubtless appear that their temperature might be sufficiently reduced to cause local precipitation in the shape of light rains, mists, and heavy dews. Continuing our line of reasoning a single step further: recalling how forests raise the degree of saturation of the air under their shadow, as well as of the adjacent atmosphere on all sides, also the well-known fact that the moist air discharges its vapor more easily in the form of rain than a dryer atmosphere, we may be pardoned for drawing the inference that warm currents sweeping over a region of country and mingling with the moist air overhanging and surrounding the woodland, would have at least a portion of the atmospheric moisture condensed into gentle showers, shedding their enlivening influences over the neighboring landscape for a considerable distance. By increasing the frequency of light rains during the vegetative season forests tend to obviate droughts, which result is of the highest importance to the farmers' crops, the climate, and all growing vegetation. Our deductions, it is seen, have been drawn largely from the known facts of observation. Forests produce abundant dews. The formation of this substance depends upon two conditions,—namely, the radiation from objects near the earth, and a certain per centum of atmospheric moisture. As in the case of the production of rain, so in the case of dew, it is more easily formed in a moist than in a dry atmosphere, the former requiring less reduction of temperature; hence, when the additional moisture in the vicinity of the forest comes in contact with the night air, dew in abundance is frequently the result. There is nothing to oppose the view that the cooler atmosphere of the shade of the grove is a source of dew during the day under certain favorable conditions,—the light breezes conveying their refreshing influences over the neighboring fields and into the valleys round about. When it is remembered that in some portions of our globe—Egypt and Arabia, for example—nearly all of the moisture reaching the earth is in the shape of dew, the reader will grant that this is no mean office on the part of sylvan nature.

Historically examining the question, it is found that there is no little conflict of evidence, though the weight of scientific opinion is strongly in favor of the doctrine that local precipitation is somewhat favored by plantations. And although in past ages the subject has been freely discussed by scientific writers of the widest fame, any inferences which do not rest upon the results of actual observations having for their object the framing of a comparison between the rainfall of wooded and unwooded districts under otherwise similar conditions, are unreliable.

In this connection the experiments of L. Fantiat and A. Sartiaux, before quoted, should be kept in remembrance. It will be recollected that the total rainfall for six months was 192.50 mm. in the forest and 177 mm. in the open air, the difference being 15.15 mm. in favor of the forest. In an interesting paper on the "Sanitary Value of Forests" (Transactions of American Public Health Association, vol. iv. pp. 56, 57), Dr. G. L. Andrews remarks: "Two points of observation have been established in Prussia, one over a young forest of Pinus sylvestris, some forty feet high, and the other over a bare, sandy plain three hundred metres distance from the edge of a woods, and at the same height from the ground. Twelve months' observation showed that, of the total rainfall within that period, ten per cent. more fell over the trees than over the bare sands three hundred feet from the trees. Experiments of a similar nature over woods of oak and beech gave an excess of five per cent. only in favor of the wooded site. Further, the mean state of the saturation of the air over the wood was ten per cent. higher than that over the bare expanse of sand, the former holding much more water in suspension than the latter (*Biederman's Centralblatt*)." Among the most trustworthy observations on this head, according to Professor J. T. Rothrock (Michaux Botanical Lectures, September 10, 1884), are those of Sir Gustav Wex, who asserts that in the Rhine, the Danube, the Elbe, the Vistula, and the Oder, the average depth of water is diminishing, and this unfortunate change he attributes to the destruction of the forests.

During 1876 the lines of equal rainfall throughout the State of Iowa (as shown by the weather report) corresponded with the lines of equal areas of woods, —the districts having the greater ratio of woodland receiving the greater precipitation. According to M. Woeikoff (*Mittheilung, loc. cit.*), at Nancy, in France, documents which show that the vicinity of the forest increases the rainfall have been collected.

Contrary opinion of a sort which can scarcely be seriously questioned has also received support. Thus, Professor J. T. Rothrock argues that it can be shown that in a number of places in this country the rainfall has increased in the last twenty years, notwithstanding the destruction of the forests. Perhaps from all the ascertainable facts of observation we are not at present warranted in affirming positively that forest-growth has the power of increasing the actual annual rainfall. And it will be remembered that such a view has not here been contended for; but, on the other hand, from the great array of facts which have been amply verified both from speculative premises and by our experiments, as well as those recorded by other competent scientific observers, certain meteorological influences may with certainty be attributed to forests, namely, that they preserve not only a higher degree of saturation of the air in their vicinity, but also a more uniform proportion of moisture than is found elsewhere; they also greatly increase the dew-fall, produce heavy mists, and by promoting the frequency of gentle showers and light rains decrease proportionately the frequency of the occurrence of drought, of heavy rains, and the ravages of torrents.

As before intimated, under their own shadow and for some distance beyond their borders, within certain limits of time, they also increase the precipitation, and this effect being more strongly manifest during summer, when the danger from drought is greater than in winter, the signal value of their effect to equalize the distribution of the rainfall will, to the mind of the reader, be free from all doubt.

Forests produce ozone. This proposition is founded upon careful observations which have been given in Chapter VI. The reader will, it is hoped, also recall the prominent part played by ozone in the removal of the organic impurities most generally found in the atmosphere. Since ozone is generated by odorous foliage and all of the flowering species, *though, the reader will remember, with greater energy by scented flowers*, the high importance to public health of the proper distribution of forests and trees is obviously apparent. Primitive nature has attended to this matter in a truly admirable fashion, but the unsparing hand of man has in many places exercised his power to the end of producing marked deterioration of climate, and in no direction has greater, though unexpected, mischief resulted than in the annihilation of one of nature's chief sources of ozone,—the forests. Some compensation for this is, however, brought about by the more general tilling of the soil following the destruction of primitive woods. In temperate climates during the winter season ordinary forests do not develop any of this substance, and this fact is measurably confirmed by the results of the recent careful researches by Dr. Nicholson (Michigan Health Board Report), who found ozone more abundant in pine-forests than in the open country in summer, and less abundant in winter. As has been shown by our researches, the exhalations from the Coniferæ evince greater energy in developing ozone than other species of forest-growth, and the present, in view of this fact, affords the writer the opportunity of entering a seasonable plea for the more careful preservation and cultivation of our American pines. Happily, these resinous species may, by proper attention to cultivation, be easily continued if the presence of certain favorable conditions of soil or climate are securable. The performance of the ozone-generating function being to a less degree under the control of the temperature than of the action of the direct rays of the sun, it follows that vegetable life and odoriferous foliage are everywhere engaged in the noble task of atmospheric purification by the agency of ozone, which, even at low temperature, is unceasingly generated, if we except periods of stormy weather. The constant action of out-door vegetation displayed in this process, it may logically be inferred, has, in divine ordination for its object the maintenance of the needful distribution and supply of atmospheric ozone. Observations such as these, if they be true, also explain the grateful purpose for which our wellnigh limitless species of wild-flowers, everywhere present, and in many cases occupying the most obscure places on the face of the earth, are designed by an all-wise Providence. Indeed, the discovery of the fact that the Floral Empire is one of the chief sources of that depurating material—without which man's struggle for life would be a struggle indeed—furnishes new import to other facts which before were utterly meaningless. We now recognize why plants in one or other quarter of the globe are in flower not only every day in the year, but, stranger still, wellnigh every hour in the day also. Thus we have "morning-glories that welcome the rising sun; chicories, dandelions, and others that wait for the rising until after breakfast. Some, like portulaccas, opuntias, and night-blooming cereus, with other plants, attend on the students who burn the midnight oil."

From the actual analysis of the beneficial effects of the two physiological functions of forests, namely, transpiration and ozonification, it may be truthfully said that their organic processes are shown to be capable of sanitary influences whose significance surpasses our most reasonable expectations. The climatic effects of forests, in all of the aspects considered, do not extend to any great distance beyond their own borders, or, in other words, their effects are chiefly local in character; hence to derive the full benefit of which they are capable it is absolutely necessary that they should be universally present in adequate proportion, and that some attention should be paid to their local distribution.

The number and particular trend of the mountain ranges, the effect of commercial intercommunication between different countries, the action of the wind, the presence of extensive bodies of water, and the absence of agriculture in unwooded districts, have in great measure determined the extent and arrangement of our forest-growth. At present writing this phase of the subject does not concern us, however.

CHAPTER X.

Natural tendency after clearing to replace old with new forest species—Difference between native species of the Atlantic and Pacific coasts—Their adaptation to conditions of soil and climate—Best proportion of woodland for sanitary objects—The forests of the United States—They need not now excite grave apprehensions—Need of better management of our forests—Arbor-day—Æsthetic influences of the woodland flora—The sanitary effects of forests—Their value at health stations—Forest air beneficial in the treatment of bronchial affections and phthisis—Climatic requisites for pulmonary invalids—The equable humidity of forests not objectionable—The advantages of pine-groves to the consumptive—Commoner forms of phthisis briefly described—The proper forest area adapted to their treatment—Suitable localities for winter and summer forest resorts—Hygienic influences of city parks—Kinds of trees for planting in streets and public parks.

CLOSELY united with the last topic alluded to in the previous chapter is the question as to what particular species are best adapted to various conditions of soil and climate. While space forbids me to discuss fully this point, it may be noted that there are few difficulties in the way of cultivating a variety of both deciduous and resinous species, more especially throughout the temperate zone, if, as will hereafter appear, we give some attention to proper cultivation, the kinds formerly native to the region in which it is desired to plant, and so forth.

Fortunately for the interests of humanity, there is an intrinsic tendency in nature to replace, without delay, the forest-growth that has been cleared away, which tendency rises to the dignity of a natural law, though frequently there is an alternation of growth, new species replacing the old. In his excellent treatise, "Man and Nature" (*loc. cit.*, pp. 27, 28), the late Mr. G. P. Marsh, after calling attention to the fact that at the commencement of the seventeenth century the soil of the North American continent, which has been occupied by British colonization, was covered with forests, with a few insignificant exceptions, tells us that whenever the Indian, in consequence of war or exhaustion of the beasts of the chase, abandoned the narrow field he had planted and the woods he had burned over, they speedily returned, by a succession of herbaceous, arborescent, and arboreal growths, to their original state. Even a single generation sufficed to restore almost to their primitive luxuriance the forest species. He further alludes to the well-known practical illustration of the same truth in the following expressive terms: "The great fire of Miramichi in 1825, probably the most extensive and terrific conflagration recorded in authentic history, spread its ravages over nearly six thousand square miles, chiefly of woodland, and was of such intensity that it seemed to consume the very soil itself. But so great was the recuperative power of nature that in twenty-five years the ground was covered again with trees of fair dimensions, except where cultivation and pasturage kept down the forest growth." On comparing the native timber species adjacent to the Atlantic coast with those of the Pacific border, however, we find they differ greatly, while the forest-growth of the Atlantic States is composed largely of those species found in Canada, on the eastern coast of Asia, and the islands of Japan; indeed, to mention the numerous species found in the Atlantic region would be to mention nearly all the species of the other regions last named. On the Pacific there are to be found but few species which flourish on the Atlantic coast. In his treatise on the "Elements of Forestry," (pp. 84, 85), Dr. Franklin B. Hough, in discussing the differences and resemblances in the native timber-growth of different regions of the United States, observes: "The Himalaya region of Northern China and Mantchuria contains many native species that may be cultivated successfully in the ornamental plantations in our Atlantic States, and are already obtainable from our great nurseries. It is already ascertained that they have better prospects of success than most of the species that thrive so remarkably in their native localities upon the Pacific coast, and under a climate and in conditions that we cannot furnish for them in the Atlantic States. They are accustomed to heavy winter rains and long, dry summers, and must have them.

"The same difficulty occurs when we attempt to cultivate on the Pacific coast many of the species that thrive in the Atlantic States. The hemlock, spruce, Norway spruce, and Australian pine among conifers, and the sugar-maple and the hickory among deciduous kinds, grow but slowly there. The pecan and the beech do better, but the locust-tree is not at all reliable." To aid to determine the kinds of trees best adapted to a given locality, he further offers this seasonable hint: "It is well to observe what kinds have grown up, or that still remain in the native growth along the borders of streams, or in places where they have been sheltered and protected."

The interrogation, What is the proper percentage of timber land to the total area for hygienic purposes? for a variety of reasons of leading practical import here needs to be answered. Thus, the destruction of the primitive forests has not been, and is not alone, for the purpose of maintaining the lumbering trade, but to a great extent, where the soil is tillable, to bring it under cultivation by the thrifty husbandman. Nor should such an encroachment upon wooded regions be discouraged, if the bounds of prudence be not overstepped.

In America, rapid increase in the population in recent times, coupled with an almost proportionate increase in the extent of interest taken in the noble calling of scientific agriculture, are circumstances which are continually creating a demand for more tillable soil, and explain why forests have been so largely invaded.

Under these circumstances, the folly of allowing to stand more forest-growth than is necessary for climatic objects, though less notable, is equally certain, notwithstanding.

In accordance with the well-proved sanitary influences previously set forth, the writer ventures to restate the proper ratio of woodland for hygienic purposes to be not less than twenty-five per centum. This should be the minimum proportion of woodland, save perhaps in the rarest conditions, or only when the natural advantages of climate prevailing in any given region are exceptional. As before intimated, to obtain their benefits in the highest degree, due regard must be paid to the question of equal distribution, which, with respect to the unwooded soil, especially in the case of cultivated regions, must be carefully considered, and is to be in great measure determined by the direction of the prevailing winds, the probable existence of malaria near by, the presence of lower or higher elevations and their particular trend, and so on. A recent writer, Mr. Chamberlain, in the *Century Magazine* (vol. xxxi. p. 535), alludes to the plains of Hungary, which " were, within a recent geological period, a desert. They are now almost unwatered save by streams from the mountains which traverse them. The water in the wells and occasional pools is very brackish, and great sand-storms even now sometimes fill the streets of Debrezzin and Pesth. Yet these plains are the most fruitful regions of Austria-Hungary, producing the richest crops of grain. They are treeless and always have been, but nature has reclaimed them." It should be observed that these plains are intermediate between mountain ranges, which operate to protect them from the effects of drying winds and other objectionable influences. As will be seen hereafter, at health stations a high ratio is frequently desirable. In the case of precipitous mountain slopes whose soil cannot be tilled, their forest covering should, if not already denuded, remain untouched, not only for the favorable effects this has upon the climate, but also in view of the fact that clearing under such circumstances is followed by destructive torrents and immeasurable damage to the surface soil. Similarly, when situated at the head-waters of streams, more especially when, as frequently occurs, these have their origin at the foot of mountainous elevations, forests are of incalculable value to promote their permanance, for reasons before mentioned, and should, when practicable, be preserved in greater abundance than indicated by the above formula. Regarding the proportionate area of forest-growth existing in America at the present time, it should be stated that while a number of States have adequate forests in good form, there are others which, though the total percentage of woodland they contain is high enough, lack that judicious proportionment that is necessary to the accomplishment of their best climatic influences. As for Pennsylvania, although containing about twenty-five per centum of forest land, there are large tracts being cultivated, more especially in hilly districts, where the local proportion of forest-growth is inadequate and constantly lessening, with evil consequences both to soil and climate. Throughout some of the Western States there appears to be dawning a lamentable paucity of forests,—a state of things which has not as yet excited grave apprehensions, however, for the future fruitfulness of these regions. Indeed, it has been argued that there are to-day more trees in the prairie States than at any previous epoch, but either as an orchard of trees, or trees planted for ornamental purposes, it must be borne in mind, they do not possess the climatic influences of a true forest, though they are not without obvious sanitary advantages. It is also doubtful whether irrigation, so extensively practised throughout Colorado and some adjacent States, would be compensation for the beneficial influences obtained from forest-trees, if we except level expanses of country, or valleys having conspicuously favorable conditions of climate. It is equally certain that, for various reasons before mentioned, in hilly agricultural places, the happy effect of a forest could not be replaced by any of the best possible devices of the human mind. Happily, the mountain ranges, extending as they do from the northern to the southern boundary lines of our country, are yet covered with a luxuriance of forest species. This is more strikingly the case in many of the Southern States, where are to be found the extensive forests of the uplands, composed for the most part of white and yellow pine, with some cypress, and amounting to not less than fifty per centum of the total acreage. Leaving these regions and travelling northward, the forests rather rapidly decrease. But if we dismiss a few Northern and Western States, the present proportion of forest area does not afford just cause for serious alarm on account of threatening evils, provided that their future ruthless destruction can be effectually checked. In view of the facts before adduced to show the strong tendency in nature to replace old with new forest vegetation, and the facility with which new forests can be grown if reasonable attention be paid to natural adaptation of the different species to soil and climate, there could be no more convincing proof to establish the truth that the best proportion of woodland area and the most desirable distribution are matters entirely within human control. What is more urgently needful is a legislative enactment that will insure the promotion of systematic sylviculture worthy of the name, or the same object might be attained still more successfully by the appointment of a competent forestry commission in each State with a view of securing better management of their individual forests.*

---

* The writer is aware of certain laws having been made which have in some degree encouraged forest-culture and tree-planting.

The latter course has recently been adopted by the State of New York, with much promise of effecting valuable work. The wisdom of the maintenance of a fair ratio of forest-growth, even though this should imply coercive policies, has from no other quarter received stronger evidence than is afforded by their climatic and sanitary advantages as herein presented. Of all national problems, there is none other for whose solution an enlightened public sentiment is so definitely valuable.

Fortunately, as indicative of the future prospect for a greater diffusion of the sort of knowledge intended to show the need of further forest legislation, it should be noted that within a comparatively recent period forest societies have been organized in this country, having for their object the discussion of interesting questions relating to the general subject; and to promote the same end it is pleasing to make mention that a periodical devoted exclusively to forestry is regularly issued. As a matter of fact, however, nearly all other nations on the globe, notably Germany, Austria, and Russia, are far in advance of America in regard to the extent and variety of their forest literature, and in the extent of attention consecrated to the interests of this important branch of science; thus, outside of our own borders, schools of forestry are, according to Hough ("Elements of Forestry," pp. 107, 108), to be found in Austria, Denmark, Finland, Germany, France, Italy, Russia, Spain, Switzerland, Sweden, and other countries. Surely, with such facts before us, the lesson for our own government is of the plainest character. As a means of encouraging the more general planting of trees, the recent introduction of so-called "Arbor-Day" by Governor Morton, of Nebraska, is deserving of elaborate mention. As evidencing the high degree of favor with which this project was received by the citizens of his State, we are told that "in the first year of its adoption more than ten million trees were planted." The custom, it is well to note, rapidly spread to the neighboring prairie States and Territories, whence it has travelled with unbroken march towards the East, having been adopted by Michigan, Ohio, and later by Pennsylvania, and already there is a grand total of seventeen States that celebrate its observance.

From the various climatic and terrestrial influences of forest-growth that have been considered, it is quite clear that they exert a potent influence upon the salubrity and healthfulness of a locality. The woodland air is highly invigorating, as evidenced by the happy results from camp life to the weary and to "run-down" subjects leading an active nomadic life among our forests at low or moderate elevations, and thus the results from practical experience agree entirely with what would be expected from our positive knowledge of the character of forest air.

"Forest-trees and plantations have an æsthetic influence. The impressions they make upon the organs of sense serve admirably to relieve mental tension, and to agreeably entertain the mind." ("Sanitary Influences of Forest Growth," address before the Philadelphia Social Science Association, Jan. 29, 1885, by the author.) Having in the former chapters experimentally shown how forests affect local climatology, particularly the hydrology of a region, it logically follows that in conditions of ill health requiring for their treatment a measurably humid air, forests in proper proportions would afford a pleasant means to attain the end desired, and they would do their work in an admirable manner. If to the above be added the fact that the air of the wilderness is charged with principles possessing therapeutic properties, and contains that highly-diligent agent, ozone, it must, it is quite obvious, be capable of rendering valuable service in connection with health stations. Owing to the opinions put forward by the writer in Chapter VII. relative to the hygienic uses of house-plants both as preventives and as remedial agents during the progress of certain diseases, it would be but natural to expect that forests hold out the same chances of relief to invalids suffering from the different forms of phthisis and other complaints who go to the numerous health resorts in search of new life and vigor. In the same chapter the probable utility of growing plants in cases of acute and chronic forms of laryngitis and bronchitis was pointed out, and for parallel reasons the atmosphere of the locality having a proportionate per centum of forest-trees rightly located can be little less effective for good during the period of vegetable growth, provided that the temperature is tolerable. For the treatment of such, the highly ozonized and terebinthinized atmosphere of the pine-groves would perhaps be preferable, more especially in cases of bronchorrhœa, in which a comparatively dry atmosphere would at least accomplish the greatest degree of comfort, if a cure be out of the question. These subjects should also make choice of well-sheltered localities, though active exercise is by no means to be interdicted. In estimating the value of the wilderness air in these cases, we should not lose sight of the supreme advantage of the changed and purified air of the forest, to wit, that it is continual in its local action on the diseased mucous membranes. If preferable, the victim of any of the forms of chronic bronchitis would receive benefit during the summer season from a trial of the most convenient forest resort. During the winter, equally good service is to be expected from the home sanitarium, such as above described.

The climatic requisites for a consumptive invalid, the reader will remember, are by most recent writers considered to be dryness, equability, and pureness. Of these, none, in the opinion of the writer, is of higher importance than the latter, namely, purity; and from the facts demonstrated by previous researches into the functions of transpiration and the generation of ozone by the forest, it may be inferred we have here the conditions most favorable to atmospheric purification. Doubtless, much of the benefit derived by patients at high altitudes is ascribable to greater purity of the air at these places than at lower levels. Forests can be shown also to favor greatly the quality of equability, both as to temperature and relative humidity. How they intercept and temper the bleak winds of winter in cold latitudes, and how by their shade and their surfaces they afford a cooler temperature in summer, has been already explained, and in this connection the importance of this influence is to be especially noted. The increase in the degree of saturation under their shade and on their environs also tends to cool the atmosphere of summer, and the unvarying degree of moisture they maintain in their vicinity are qualities which in the highest degree favor an equable clime. They should be favorably situated with respect to prevailing winds, or marshy localities which are known to cause malaria frequently. With respect to the degree of moisture in the climatic management of phthisis, there is great diversity of opinion, though undeniably the majority of the best authorities have pronounced in favor of dry climes. Just here it is well to note how unfortunate for science that to the term "dry air" is given such an unparalleled latitude of meaning. "Writers have the habit of speaking of the atmosphere as dry, when in reality it contains considerable moisture. For example, the air of Atlantic City is spoken of as dry and bracing, as is also that of Denver, Colorado. Now, let any one take the meteorological reports of those places for the five winter months ending with March, as the writer has done, and reckon from Glaisher's table their absolute humidity. It will be found that the former place has nearly twice as much by weight of vapor per cubic foot of atmosphere as the latter." ("The Relation of Forests to Health Resorts," *Philadelphia Medical Times*, May 20, 1882, by the author.)

But, as indicated and pointed out in a previous chapter, it is not my design to contest the fact that certain invalids, particularly some cases of chronic phthisis, in whom a good degree of strength is retained and who are yet in the earlier stages of the affection, are not greatly benefited or even apparently cured by a prolonged residence at high altitude where the air is quite dry. The reader will remember how large a class of consumptive invalids is composed on the one hand of those who cannot bear the expense of making a prolonged change to such a resort, and on the other those in whom the condition of the patient is unsuited to a high elevation. In the latter category it will be remembered we have placed those in the last stage of the disease; those cases which are rapidly progressive with or without frequent hæmoptysis; those patients who are excessively weak, while the local lesions may be quite slight; and finally those having a highly-sensitive nervous system, or in whom there is a morbid susceptibility of the mucous membrane to the action of extreme cold, all of whom cannot endure the severity of a bleak clime, such as obtains in Colorado, for example. Probably the cases usually regarded as being best adapted to dry climes would do equally well if they were to repair to a resort where forests abound at about six thousand feet elevation. But it has been urged against this view by certain writers that since forests increase the local humidity, they are objectionable at such resorts. Whatever objections may be opposed to moisture derived from other sources, there are certain indisputable facts going to show that a fair degree of humidity derived from forest flora is generally valuable to consumptives, partly because it is very nearly uniform, and partly because, as has been pointed out, it is widely different from ordinary moisture, having undergone marked change by passing through plants. If, however, a low forest humidity be desirable, this is attainable by attention to the ratio of woodland to the general surface. It should be specially observed that the beneficial influences of forests growing out of the function of transpiration and the generation of ozone are equally as potent at a low as at a higher temperature, provided that the weather be clear. In colder climes, Minnesota, for example, which are definitely serviceable to a certain class of consumptives, forests exercise a potent sanitary influence in tempering bleak winds, thus affording shelter under their estuaries, and in modifying extremes of temperature. The equable humidity of forests would also insure less variable temperature than the same degree of ordinary moisture,—a fact of great significance to consumptive invalids in cold and severe climes. Hence in the latter clime it would appear evident forests, for such reasons alone, would be most trustworthy adjuncts at health stations. Moreover, by strict attention to the character of vegetation, the percentage of woodland, and elevation, a nearly exact degree of saturation desirable can be obtained. To illustrate, at a resort of medium or high altitude not more than fifty per cent. of forest area would produce the effect suited to the cases demanding a comparatively dry clime, since the small increase of humidity thereby occasioned would be vastly more than counterbalanced by other beneficial influences exercised by the forests. From the structural peculiarities of the pine-leaves being dense and having a thick cuticular covering, the function of transpiration is carried on at about one-third of the rate which takes place from forest-trees having soft, thin leaves. Hence the effect of pine-forests upon the degree of saturation of the atmosphere is very slight, and they can scarcely be said to be open to the same objections in this regard as forests composed of deciduous species. Thus pine-forests situated upon a mountain six thousand feet high would increase the natural advantages of the climate by their emanations, more particularly the abundance of ozone they are capable of generating. Rhone Mountain, to which allusion will hereafter be made, represents a resort such as above depicted.

We also find them on passing in a northerly direction from the latter place, especially through some of the Western States.

Having now sufficiently discussed the element of humidity in general and the relation of forest moisture thereto, in order to arrive at conclusions which are to be reliable in the choice of a resort modified by forest exhalations, it will be necessary further to distinguish, from a clinical point of view, between some of the commoner forms of phthisis, and to indicate approximately the extent and character of the forest vegetation best adapted to them severally.

"Perhaps the majority of cases of phthisis develop very gradually, the only symptom at first being slight cough, which attracts little or no attention. By and by there is slight expectoration, the appetite fails, the pulse is quickened, and bodily strength diminishes. These symptoms persist and become intensified, with feverish excitement and perceptible falling off in flesh. Frequently about this period the doctor is consulted, and on making a physical exploration of the chest finds evidence of the commencement of pathological changes in the lungs so characteristic of the disease in question.

"There is a catarrhal form of consumption with inflammatory action, implicating the bronchial and laryngeal mucous membranes, originating usually in cold, raw climes. Another form of the disease is known as laryngeal phthisis, in which the chief difficulty rests with the larynx." ("Relations of Forests to Health Resorts," *loc. cit.*)

The above kinds of cases, particularly the first, when not attended by marked hectic fever and not far advanced with regard to the lesions of the lungs, or, to speak more accurately, when still in the earlier stages of the affection, would receive great benefit from the woodland air in mountainous districts. Having seen that the beneficial effect of forests is but local, the patient should, when practicable, keep somewhere near by the forests, or, better still, within their shelter, thus giving the vapors and the ozone which emanate from the trees an opportunity to perform their continuous gentle atomization and aid in forwarding good results. Additionally, the air of the wilderness also benefits by promoting sleep, increasing the appetite, and improving nutrition, the latter effect being doubtless attributable to the action of the ozone upon the human system. Here are two truths which are to be observed, if we wish to obtain the most successful results. The soil of the woodland should always be dry, with little vegetable mould, and should be *non-malarious;* and the earlier the patient is sent to his new refuge *the better.* The region should afford a forest area of about fifty per centum. The degree of elevation and the character of the particular climate selected must be largely determined by the degree of strength retained, and the other peculiarities of the condition of individual patients, the object here being to give merely a general idea of the proportion of woods and the character of climate suited to some of the commoner forms of consumption. There are in the United States numerous delightful resorts suitable for the above category of patients, both during the summer and the winter seasons. These are to be found through the Northwestern States of Minnesota, Wisconsin, and Colorado, or, starting from the northern coast line and passing southerly, we meet with them in New York, where are to be found in magnificent form the Adirondacks, in Pennsylvania, whose grand old Alleghanies afford a goodly number, in Virginia, and through the Carolinas. If his strength does not disallow of it, a patient suffering from any one of the conditions above outlined should lead an active nomadic life, making frequent woodland excursions, since, to realize the greatest benefit from the forest air, exercise is essential. In the category of cases above described there is a large element whose conditions call for a comparatively dry, pure atmosphere, and hence such should, if strength will admit of it, and the disease is not rapidly progressing, seek the higher eminences. An elevation of from four thousand to six thousand feet, with fifty per centum of forests, would be peculiarly appropriate. For such conditions pine-groves would, for reasons before intimated, be preferable. The value of the latter has had numerous advocates, among which occurs the name of the famous New York physician, Professor A. Loomis, in whose opinion camping in the pine-forests is exceedingly valuable to consumptive invalids. There is an excellent example of such a climate in North Carolina, where pine-forests are so highly-favorably situated, namely, Rhone Mountain, which has an elevation of six thousand three hundred and ninety-four feet, and is covered with vegetation almost to its summit. The species found near the base of the mountain are the walnut, oak, maple, gum, poplar, magnolia, and others, while at the higher points evergreens, spruces, and pines abound. As before stated, there are no facts to oppose the practice of sending these subjects to forest resorts in the colder climates of Minnesota, Wisconsin, and other adjacent States.

There is another large class of consumptive invalids, before incidentally alluded to, demanding a moister and milder climate than that above described. They include nearly all cases of phthisis of whatever form who are far advanced, or have reached what is termed by medical writers the third or last stage of the disease, with extensive morbid changes of the lungs. At this stage the chiefest symptoms are great weakness and emaciation, troublesome cough, difficulty in breathing, night-sweats, loss of appetite, and sometimes diarrhœa. To this category also belong the patients in whom there is no correlation between the almost complete loss of general strength and the small portion of the lung implicated, as well as those cases occurring chiefly among females, who are possessed of a highly-sensitive nervous system, or whose bronchial mucous membranes are exceedingly susceptible to the vicissitudes of temperature. For the latter classes to resort to high altitudes or to unusually cold climates would be gross folly, and for them to attempt to lead a nomadic life would only too soon result in aggravation of their condition. On the contrary, they need a genial clime to invite them out of doors, with more or less humidity of the air, according to the peculiarities of the disease and individual, encircling the feverish frame, which state of air often renders great service in contributing to the patient's comfort,—an office not to be despised in these usually hopeless cases. For this class of sufferers, the districts to which they are sent should afford not less than seventy-five per cent. of forest-growth. The relative per centum would also be naturally determined to a great extent by the proximity of the resort to the coast and the degree of elevation. The air of such a forest resort does good service in alleviating urgent symptoms, such as troublesome cough, irritability of the nervous system, intensity of the hectic flush, and so on, and thus it aids in delaying, if not arresting, the onward progress of the disease to a fatal issue. The reader will recall the fact that our home sanitarium described in the previous chapter holds out chances of successful treatment in this class of cases, during the cold season. Should, however, the invalid of this class be not too far removed, and should he retain some degree of strength, he might make trial of one of the numerous examples of winter forest resorts adapted to the treatment of cases of this description, which resorts are to be found throughout some of our Southern States, particularly South Carolina and Georgia. Starting at Aiken, South Carolina, latitude about 33° 5′, and passing in a southeast direction until Thomasville, Georgia, is reached, latitude 30° 5′, at an elevation varying from five hundred to two thousand feet, where flourish the pine-forests above alluded to in abundance. Already at various places along these mountain ranges there are to be seen many health stations, and among them we may mention Mount Airy and Eastman's, near Macon, South Carolina, and Thomasville, in Southern Georgia, which latter has numerous advocates in the medical profession, and as it has an elevation of only about five hundred feet, in a mild and charming climate, with ample pine-forests, it is peculiarly suited for meeting the indications of the class of invalids under discussion. The above places, which, however, have been brought in recent times to the notice of the profession, have proved to be exceedingly operative in their good effects upon pulmonary invalids when the cases have been properly chosen. It is a fact of practical observation that consumptives are abandoning the low, moist places on the Florida coasts, while the popular tide has been of late tending towards the pine-forests of the uplands. Here also the soil is dry and sandy; the atmosphere contains considerable humidity, is impregnated with the balsamic vapors from the pines, which furnish sufficient ozone for purposes of atmospheric purification, and the further purpose of effecting favorable changes in the blood of the patient. To consumptive invalids, according to the entire experience of those who have made this climate their temporary refuge, the air is strikingly agreeable and bracing. Numerous instances have been reported to the medical periodicals by physicians exhibiting the value of a residence at these health resorts.

Having pointed out measures and appropriate localities for the second class of invalids during the winter, it remains to be queried, Where shall they go during the warm season? In the first place, should the patient be living in a climate whose midsummer temperature is not objectionably high, we deem it free from doubt that he could do no better, especially if he be living in a rural district and a flower-lover, than to remain at home, and engage in the health-giving enterprise of the culture of plants both in-doors and out. And for the sake of change he might, if conveniently located, spend some of his hours in the neighboring forest. And when, as is usual in most latitudes, the summer heat, and especially in large cities, is great and quite injurious in its tendency, the question of change of air meets us fairly. Without detaining the reader with a description of special places, there are doubtless forest resorts not far from every large city throughout the temperate zone, and this is particularly true of the wooded hills and mountain ranges of our own Keystone. In our own latitude of Philadelphia, any of the forests near by would be all that could be desired for the present class. The places selected should, of course, possess certain natural elements regarding topographic arrangement and surrounding scenery. The soil, as already intimated, should be dry, and hotel accommodation of the best. The present group of sufferers being greatly debilitated, and having extensive lesions of the lungs, do not usually retain sufficient strength to allow of an active, roving life among hills and mountain ranges, and hence they should lead a more quiet existence at a lower level and at places well sheltered from strong winds. If the invalid be unaccustomed to a varied social life, a residence at some farm-house, properly located with respect to the surrounding forests, affording a good *cuisine* and other home comforts, would answer his every purpose. The patient should spend as much time as possible in the shadow of the woods, and for such there ought to be opportunity for short excursions in the environs. During the hottest season, such subjects would find densely-shaded nooks, owing to their decidedly lower temperature, add greatly to their convenience and physical comfort. In my opinion it is an especially important truth that the sufferer from consumption belonging to the second class depicted should not undertake to reach noted resorts a long distance away, and this chiefly for two reasons: first, they can receive equal benefits nearer home, and, secondly, long journeys in these debilitated subjects are always attended by injurious consequences on their advent. The practice of expatriation under these circumstances is, to put it mildly, almost cruel. The air of the woodland is highly beneficial in run-down conditions from other causes, and during convalescence from many acute diseases. Upon the authority of Dr. Oswald (*Popular Science Monthly* for August, 1877), scirrhous affections of the skin disappear under the disinfecting influences of the forest air. He also quotes Dr. Brehm, who has observed that ophthalmia and leprosy, which have become hereditary diseases not only in the valley of the Nile, but also in the table lands of Barca and Tripoli, are utterly unknown in the well-timbered valley of Abyssinia, though the Abyssinians live more than a hundred geographical miles nearer to the equator than their afflicted neighbors.

SANITARY INFLUENCES OF FOREST-GROWTH.

Since our city parks and public squares may be regarded as forests of reduced size, it will appear obvious to the reader that they also are capable of valuable hygienic influences. The writer having elsewhere ("Sanitary Influences of Forest-Growth," *loc. cit.*, pp. 13, 14) called brief attention to their beneficial effects upon the air of cities, his remarks are here quoted: "It must be confessed that nowhere could trees and ornamental shrubbery prove their virtues to greater advantage to the public health than by improving the conditions of a vitiated city atmosphere. As in the case of forests, the action of public grounds must needs be of a local character; hence it is quite obvious that in large cities quite a number of squares of the size of those in Philadelphia would be needed to produce the desired effect. The conclusions respecting the influence of forests upon local climate apply, with few exceptions of little importance, in the present instance. For obvious reasons, their effect in mitigating the extremes of temperature by checking the force of wind currents is here almost negative, but the trees, by causing refreshing shade and transpiring aqueous vapor, have a delightful cooling effect, thus tending to moderate oppressive midsummer heat of our large cities. Along with the moist vapors constantly emitted there are also other health-giving principles evolved, and among them ozone is perhaps the most important. Since only the flower and odoriferous foliage are ozone-generating, the vegetation of these public parks should be selected with due regard to this fact. The same percentage of the total area should be assigned for retreats of this kind as was indicated when speaking of the proper ratio of woodland for ordinary sanitary purposes, namely, twenty-five. But what city can boast of such a percentage of forest area?" Perhaps the city affording a forest area approaching most nearly to this standard is Cleveland, Ohio, which has been happily termed "The Forest City," and by the side of this may be placed "The City of Elms," New Haven. "This would also be manifestly impossible in those portions of older cities already densely built up, but even here a nearer approach to the proper standard might be attained by the general planting of trees on either side of our thoroughfares. This latter suggestion, if carried out, would have the effect of improving the air of our streets, which is really the air we breathe, and thus by means of free ventilation a purer and wholesomer atmosphere would be admitted into our dwellings.

"It is quite evident that by providing sufficient reservations of this sort a perfect boon would be conferred upon that large element of our population, the humbler classes, who for financial reasons are unable to make a change of residence during the heated term. Again, such squares form a convenient substitute for a more complete change of air in the cases of that large class of little patients suffering from the infantile diseases of summer.

"Who can question but that the lives savable by the maintenance of a sufficient number of these public parks could be counted by tens of thousands? For in all medical knowledge there is no fact better established than that the usual summer ailments of infants can be most successfully treated by change of air. Than the subject of open squares and their keeping up under proper regulations, there is none more important inviting the attention of our municipal law-makers, and it is no exaggeration to say that any improvements they might make in this regard would be rewarded by a realizing sense of having done the greatest good to the greatest number."

While in recent times certain other advantages of these city parks have been pointed out, namely, their refining and educating influence; their rank as places from which solid enjoyments of life are to be drawn; their fully-appreciated beauty when artistic effect is displayed in their arrangement; their value for purposes of shade in summer, and so on, the best reasons yet presented, the reader will doubtless be willing to concede, for providing and continuing such public resorts under official administration are furnished from the side of their sanitary effects. A single word as to the particular species to be planted. For street planting it is best to select a single species for each street, and among the most suitable for this use are the maple, poplars, certain oaks, locusts, lindens, and others. In making choice of species for grounds of public resort this thought should be paramount, namely, that such resorts be made as nearly representative of the true forest as possible, if, as before incidentally stated, the greatest hygienic benefits are to be expected. Besides the kinds most usually met with in the woodland flora, the horse-chestnut and catalpas would lend additional attractiveness. In short, there should here be great diversity of species, and chiefly for the reason that this would procure a more nearly continuous supply of ozone to the air, since the various species would put forth their blossoms at different times during the period of vegetable growth. For reasons still more obvious, the resinous species should never fail to be selected for their effect in developing this active body. For rules to serve as a guide as to the best methods to be adopted in planting, the reader is referred to the hints contained in the chapter on "Practical Floriculture." He can also consult with advantage works on forestry.

Finally, it is my wish to call brief attention to the evident sanitary advantages held out by judicious planting of private grounds. As can be attested by numerous living examples, the man who engages with some degree of enthusiasm in the work of planting trees and shrubbery on his homestead achieves no slight blessing in the way of enjoyment and contentment from his new vocation, apart from the well-known hygienic benefits to be derived from such a course.

In one of the numbers (583) of the *Spectator*, Addison (quoted by Hough, *loc. cit.*, page 114) has the following: "There is indeed something truly magnificent in this kind of amusement. It gives a nobler air to several parts of nature; it fills the earth with a variety of beautiful scenes, and has something in it like creation. For this reason the pleasure of one who plants is something like that of the poet, who, as Aristotle observed, is more delighted with his productions than any other writer or artist that is known. Plantations have one advantage in them which is not to be found is most other works, as they give a pleasure of a more lasting date, and continually improve in the eye of the planter. When you have finished a building or any other undertaking of a like nature, it immediately begins to decay on your hands; you see it brought to its utmost point of perfection, and from that time hastening to its ruin. On the contrary, when you have finished your plantations they are still arriving at higher degrees of perfection as long as you live, and appear more delightful in each succeeding year than they did in the foregoing."

Though utterances such as the above show beautifully how efficacious is the practice of tree-planting to foster the interests of sylviculture, yet a knowledge of the hygienic advantages offered by these sylvan gifts of nature, which advantages the pages of this book will, it is hoped, convey to the mind of the cultivator, will scarcely fail of the effect to invest the custom with new and lively interest still better calculated to promote the same good cause.

INDEX.

Absorption, 44.
Abyssinia, 324.
Addison, 328.
Animal and vegetable worlds, functional comparisons between, 29.
Antiquatis Feralium apud Græcos et Romanos, 22.
Aquariums, 243, 244.
Arbor-Day, 311.
Aristotle, 328.
Arum, the, 79.
Assimilation, 31.
    beneficial effect of, upon respirable medium, 32.
Atlantic City, humidity of air of, 314.
Atmosphere, analysis of, from Libyan Desert, Mont Blanc, and Bengal jungles, 38.
Atomizers, Nature's, plants as, 195.
Australia, 293.

Bacillus malariæ, 62.
    tuberculosis, 177, 178.
Bacteria, 145.
    cause of zymotic diseases, 146.
Benedict, Pope, 272.
Bernard, Claude, celebrated experiments of, 29.
Bouquets, preparation and preservation of, hints regarding, 51.
Boussingault, 35.
Bronchitis, chronic, 166, 167, 168, 172.

Cailletet, 51.
Carbon dioxide, in the atmosphere of cities, 35.
    in dwellings and crowded apartments, 39.
Chlorophyll, 31.
City of Elms, the, 326.
Coniferæ, ozone-exhalations from, 301.
Conservatories, 246.
    arrangements for, 247, 248.

Consumption, tubercular, 174.
    prevalent mortality of, 175.
    etiological conditions, 176.
    infectiousness of, inferred, 176.
    demonstrated, 177, 178.
    general hygienic measures for, 190.
Consumptives, midsummer resorts for, 323.
Contaminations, atmospheric, in the house, 144, 145.
    developing fevers, 145.
Coriander, Mons., 32.
Corson, Dr. Hiram, 21.
Crudeli, Prof. Tommasi, bacteriologist, 55, 262.
Croup, true, 163.
Cuttings, fungi fatal to, 226.

Density, atmospheric, compensated by number of respirations, 42.
De Saussure, researches of, 34.
Diathermancy, 289.
Disforesting, ominousness of, 258.
Drainage, 65.
    subsoil, 262.
Dry heat, when admissible, 110.
Ducharte, observations of, 48, 218.
"Dumb Ague," 56.

Eucalyptus globulus, 263, 264.
Evaporation, from human body, 106, 107.
    soil, hindered by forest-growth, 259.
    conclusion of Ebermayer concerning, 260.
    demonstrative experiments upon, 285, 287.
    in forests, 286.
Exhalations, plant, modifying influences of, in bronchitis, 168.

Fertilizers, general, 211.
    chemical, use of, 213.
Fevers, intermittent, 57.
    remittent, how regarded, 58.

Floriculture, home, fruition of, 328.
  practical, sanitary benefits of, 184, 197.
Florida, climatic advantages of, 191.
Flowers, moral and æsthetic influences of, 147, 148, 149.
Flower-pots, 220.
  forms of, 220, 221.
  characteristic advantages, 221, 222.
  packing of, 222.
Foliage, aqueous absorption by, 52, 53.
Forest City, the, 326.
Forestry, schools of, 310.
Forests, 257.
  destruction of, 258.
  streams dependent upon, 261.
  unfavorable to malarial soil, 263.
  influence of, on rainfall, 269, 295.
  chemico-vital action of, 270.
  barriers to the spread of malarial germs, 271, 272.
  preventives of cholera, instances cited, 273, 274, 275.
  climatic effects of, 276.
  wind-currents opposed by, 277.
  protection by, from drying winds, 278.
  temperature of in summer, 279, 280.
  winter temperature of, 282.
  marked effects of, upon atmospheric humidity, 283.
  transpiration in, 284, 286.
  production of ozone by, 300.
Forest-trees, æsthetic influence of, 311.
Functions, animal and vegetable, harmony of, 22.
"Funereal plants," 22.
Fungi, microscopic, destructive action of, 233, 234.
Furnace, hot-air, 108.
  house-plants as correctives of evil results of, 108.

Gardeners, observations of, general health of, 183.
  instances cited, 183, 184, 185, 186, 187, 188.
  modern skill of, 209.
Gardening, out-door, 252.

Gardening, select plants for, 253.
  massing system in, 253, 254.
Garreau, demonstration of, 97.
Gernium, experiment upon, to determine evaporation, 48.
Germ, malarial, when innocuous, 66.
  in the soil, 87.
Greenhouse, conservatory originally distinct from, 245.
  requirements for, 249, 250.
Grosvenor Square, 16.

Hall, Horticultural, experiments in, 119, 120.
Health resorts, forest as, for phthisical cases, 315, 316, 318.
  classification of, in the United States, for consumptives, 319, 321, 322.
Henderson, Mr., floriculturist, 24.
Himalaya region, 305.
Holmes, Oliver Wendell, 18.
Hot-houses, when so termed, 250.
House-plants, efficacy of in chronic diseases, 158, 160.
  nervous lesions, 161.
  catarrhal affections, 165.
  in sick-rooms, professional indifference concerning, 182.
Humidity, atmospheric, proper standard of, 106.
  lack of, in dwellings, 106.
  uniformity of, in plants, 105.
  hygienic importance of equanimity of, 107.
Humus, consideration of, 268.

Ignorant superstition, decline of, the result of scientific observation, 25, 26.
Impurities, atmospheric, lessened by ozonizing function in plants, 147.
India, Central, incident in, 274.
Insects, ravages of, in plant-growing, 229, 232.
  means for destroying, 230, 231.
Invalids, consumptive, climatic requisites for, 313.
Irrigation, inadequacy of, 308.

"Jersey swamps," 212.

Koch, Prof., of Berlin, 177.

Lachrymal vases, 36.
Lancisci, 60.
Laryngitis, 162.

INDEX. 333

Leaf area, 284.
Lessons, two poignant, 68.
Liebig, Prof., 36.
Linnæus the naturalist, 13.
Livingstone, Dr., observations by, 292, 293.
Locke, John, 181.
London Globe, extracts from, 20.

Malaria, increased prevalence of, 56.
   popular denominations of, 57.
   symptoms of, cursorily noticed, 59.
   origin of morbific agent of, 61.
   prevalence of, at deltas and estuaries, 61.
   essential conditions for propagation of, 63.
   the cause of, a living ferment, 64.
Mariotte, experiments by, 45.
Marsh miasm, 60.
McCulloch, 64.
Miramichi, great fire of, 304.
Munich, observations at, 275.
Mythology, emblematic plants in, 23.

Nectaries, description of, 139.

Odors, disagreeable, 70.
Oil of roses, 70.
Oxygen, presence of, in assimilated substances, 31.
Ozone, 112.
   artificial generation of, 114.
   generated by growing plants and flowers, 130.
   tests for, the Schönbein and guaiacum, 115.
   marked properties of, 117, 118.
   series of observations of, 120, 121.
   apparatus devised, 124.
   out-door reactions more marked, 126, 127.
   experiments with Coleus blumei, 131, 132.
      Fuchsia globosa, 132.
      Vinca rosea, 133.
      Lilium longiflorum, 133.
      Geranium (pelargonium), 134.
      Pinus strobus, 134, 135.
      Norway spruce, 135.

Ozone, formula deduced, regarding, 136.
   tabular record of results, 137, 138, 139.
   vital influence of, on the atmosphere, 142.

Palmella, 62.
Parks, city, sanitary virtue of, 325.
Passion for flowers, Oriental, 17.
Pettenkofer, Prof. von, 16, 23, 40, 270.
   dictum of, 33.
Phthisis, a specific microbe the cause of, 177, 178, 179, 180.
   not unpreventable, 181.
   radical cure of, not assured, 180, 189.
Plant-life, proportion of, for phthisical cases, 198, 199.
Plant-respiration, earlier opinions concerning, in light and darkness, 30.
Plants, early superstition regarding, 15.
   elaborate cultivation of, conducive to artistic refinement, 16.
   absorption of moisture by, 44.
   ozone generating, in living-rooms, 143, 144.
   flowering species, the most active, 150.
   hygienic influences of, 76.
   sanitary advantages of, in sick-rooms, 154.
   cases cited, 199, 200, 201, 202, 203, 204, 205, 206, 207.
   recapitulation, 208.
   to aid, not supplant, customary medical measures, 156.
Potting, practical hints in, 223, 224, 225.
Pouchet, 16, 31.
Protoplasm, 77.
   defined, 77.
   properties of, 78.

Radiation, terrestrial, 288.
   defined, 289.
Rafflesia, 71.
Railways, construction of, attended by increased prevalence of malaria, 64.

Rainfall, observations upon the, 298, 299.
　equalized by forest-growth, 299.
Respiration, plant, 19, 32.
Rhone Mountain, 317, 320.
Roots, 216.
　effect of moisture upon, 217, 218.
　warmth upon, 219, 220.
Roscoe, 35.
Royal Winter Garden, 41.
Russian lady, singular case of, 65.

Sachs, 46.
　experiments explaining withering of plants, 47.
Salisbury, palmella or ague plant of, 62.
Sanitarium, floral, the, 191, 192.
　home, the results attainable in, 194.
Saturation, degree of, 296.
　influenced by forest-growth, 297.
Scents, bouquet, whimsicalities regarding, 73.
Schizomycete, 62.
Scott, Sir Edward, 15.
Shakespeare, quoted, 18.
Siculus, Diodorus, 72.
Soil, potting, preferences for, 210, 211.
　formula for, suggested, 210.
　special, 212.
Solarium, New York Hospital, 157.
Southern States, 321.
Southey, Mrs., quoted, 17.
Species, forest, difference between, in Atlantic and Pacific States, 304, 305.
Spectator, the, extract from, 328.
Squares, public, artistic effect of, 327.
Stillé, Prof. A., 109.
Strache, Colonel Richard, 291.
Street-planting, trees for, 327.
Suggestion, practical, to the complainant, 59.
Sylviculture, systematic, urgency of, 309.
"Systems of bottom heat," 220.

Theophrastus, 45.
Tobacco-smoke, 231.
Transpiration, 79.

Transpiration, an organic function, 79.
　discovery of, by Mueschenbroeck, 80.
　experimental labors upon, 81, 82, 83.
　experiments upon, by author, 85.
　methods employed, 85, 86, 87.
　experiments with Calla Æthiopica, 87.
　　Pelargonium cucullata, 88.
　　Fuchsia (F. macrostemma), 88, 89.
　　Hydrangea, 90.
　　Camellia japonica, 90, 91.
　　Lantana (L. carnosa), 91.
　　Dracæna, 92.
　rate of, tabulated, 93, 94, 95, 96.
　influence of sunlight in, 98.
　　wind-currents, 99.
　importance of ratio of, 100.
　hygienic conditions of the air affected by, 102.
　effect of, on the humidity of the air in dwellings, 103, 104.
　indirect effect of, in hygiene, 288.
Tuberose, 74.
Tyndall, Prof., experiments by, 271, 290.

Vapors, moist, significant importance of, in phthisis, 181.
Varieties, seed, 228.
Vegetable perfumes, ozone-converting action of, upon oxygen, 140, 141.
Vegetation, relation between, and atmospheric ozone, 130.

Washington Observatory, 272.
Water, movement of, through stems, 78.
Watery vapor, effect of, on radiant heat, 290.
　meteorological data, 291.
　observations in Australia, 293.
Window-gardeners, tools for, 244, 245.
Window-gardening, 237.
　requisites for, 239, 240, 241, 242.
Woodland, equable humidity of, 261.
　percentage of, 306.

www.ingramcontent.com/pod-product-compliance
Lightning Source LLC
Chambersburg PA
CBHW021202230426
43667CB00006B/511